PICTORIAL REVIEW OF PEDIATRICS

*Acute Care and
Emergency Medicine*

Gary R. Fleisher, M.D.
Professor of Pediatrics
Harvard Medical School
Chief, Emergency Medicine, Children's Hospital
Boston, Massachusetts

Stephen Ludwig, M.D.
Associate Physician in Chief
Children's Hospital of Philadelphia
Professor of Pediatrics
University of Pennsylvania School of Medicine
Philadelphia, Pennsylvania

Associate Authors

Marc N. Baskin, M.D.
Instructor of Pediatrics, Harvard Medical School
Senior Physician, Emergency Medicine
Service Chief, Short Stay Program
Children's Hospital
Boston, Massachusetts

Jane M. Lavelle, M.D.
Assistant Professor of Pediatrics
University of Pennsylvania School of Medicine
Senior Physician, Pediatric Emergency Medicine
Children's Hospital of Philadelphia
Philadelphia, Pennsylvania

Consulting Author

Paul K. Woolf, M.D.
Assistant Professor of Pediatrics
Associate Director
Division of Pediatric Cardiology
New York Medical College
Valhalla, New York

PICTORIAL REVIEW OF PEDIATRICS

Acute Care and Emergency Medicine

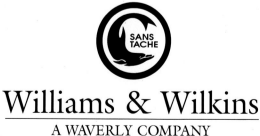

Williams & Wilkins

A WAVERLY COMPANY

BALTIMORE • PHILADELPHIA • LONDON • PARIS • BANGKOK
BUENOS AIRES • HONG KONG • MUNICH • SYDNEY • TOKYO • WROCLAW

Editor: Kathleen Courtney Millet
Managing Editor: Joyce A. Murphy
Marketing Manager: Daniell T. Griffin
Production Coordinator: Raymond E. Reter
Project Editor: Jeffrey S. Myers
Designer: Shepherd, Inc., Dubuque, Iowa
Illustration Planner: Lorraine Wrzosek
Cover Designer: Shepherd, Inc., Dubuque, Iowa
Typesetter: Maryland Composition Company, Inc., Glen Burnie, Maryland
Printer & Binder: R. R. Donnelley & Sons, Willard, Ohio
Digitized Illustrations: Maryland Composition Company, Inc., Glen Burnie, Maryland

351 West Camden Street
Baltimore, Maryland 21201-2436 USA

Rose Tree Corporate Center
1400 North Providence Road
Building II, Suite 5025
Media, Pennsylvania 19063-2043 USA

Accurate indications, adverse reactions and dosage schedules for drugs are provided in this book, but it is possible that they may change. The reader is urged to review the package information data of the manufacturers of the medications mentioned.

Printed in the United States of America

Library of Congress Cataloging-in-Publication Data

Fleisher, Gary R. (Gary Robert), 1951-
    Pictorial review of pediatrics : acute care and emergency medicine / Gary R. Fleisher, Stephen Ludwig ; associate authors, Marc N. Baskin, Jane M. Lavelle ; consulting author, Paul K. Woolf.
        p.   cm.
    Includes bibliographical references and index.
    ISBN 0-683-30267-1
    1. Pediatric emergencies—Atlases.   2. Pediatric intensive care—Atlases.   I. Ludwig, Stephen, 1945-
II. Title
    [DNLM: 1. Emergencies—in infancy & childhood—case studies.   2. Emergencies—in infancy & childhood—examination questions.   3. Diagnosis, Differential—in infancy & childhood—examination questions.   4. Critical Care—in infancy & childhood—examination questions.   WS 205 F596p 1998]
    RJ370.F63   1998
    618.92'0025—dc21
    DNLM/DLC
    for Library of Congress   97-28142
                                                                                                                              CIP

The publishers have made every effort to trace the copyright holders for borrowed material. If they have inadvertently overlooked any, they will be pleased to make the necessary arrangements at the first opportunity.

To purchase additional copies of this book, call our customer service department at **(800) 638-0672** or fax orders to **(800) 447-8438**. For other book services, including chapter reprints and large quantity sales, ask for the Special Sales department.

Canadian customers should call **(800) 665-1148**, or fax **(800) 665-0103**. For all other calls originating outside of the United States, please call **(410) 528-4223** or fax us at **(410) 528-8550**.

Visit Williams & Wilkins on the Internet: http://www.wwilkins.com or contact our customer service department at **custserv@wwilkins.com**. Williams & Wilkins customer service representatives are available from 8:30 am to 6:00 pm, EST, Monday through Friday, for telephone access.

98 99 00 01
2 3 4 5 6 7 8 9 10

PREFACE

Beginning with a fixed focus camera, progressing to an inexpensive 35 mm SLR with a set of interchangeable close-up lenses, and now using top-of-the line photographic equipment with autofocus and a ring flash, we have been taking pictures of our experiences in the emergency department for the past twenty years, as well as saving electrocardiograms and radiographs along the way. The enthusiastic response to our teaching collection, from students, residents, and practicing physicians over the past two decades, has prompted us to put together this book, which we are pleased to share with you.

We set out on this project with several goals in mind. Primarily, we believe that readers of this text will learn pediatric acute care and emergency medicine, along with a good deal of general pediatrics. Perhaps equally important, we hope to introduce or refine for clinicians an approach to thinking about patients. Whether preparing for a board examination or plowing through an ever-growing stack of specialty journals, all who embark on a career in medicine remain perpetual students. Not only do all of us need to augment our databases continually, but in addition we must sharpen our ability to dissect out relevant clinical facts efficiently in the midst of multiple, brief, and complex encounters. For all those who wish to become more knowledgeable and/or to hone their judgment, regardless of postgraduate level or specialty, this book should prove an appropriate resource.

Secondarily, we have assembled a study guide. Although not our major aim, we believe that the format which we have chosen will provide assistance to those preparing for primary board examinations as well as recertification, particularly in Pediatrics, Emergency Medicine, Pediatric Emergency Medicine, and Family Practice. Standard textbooks are wonderful, and we would be pleased to recommend at least one to you, but most physicians can read for only so long and then retain only a small fraction of any written material. We believe the combination of visual stimuli with a question-and-answer format will prove a much more successful strategy.

Finally, we want to share the excitement that each of us derives from our practices. Working in an emergency department or an office and being prepared to tackle whatever walks through the doors keeps the adrenaline pumping in many of us. We hope our presentation will mimic real life encounters closely enough so as to elicit at least a mild sympathomimetic surge, if not an actual tachycardia.

The organization of this book needs some explanation to allow for optimal utilization. While we think you will find it uniquely helpful, it is admittedly unconventional, but intentionally so. The sequence of the cases bears no relationship to the diagnoses. The pictures come to you, as do patients in practice, with a complaint or a story, rather than with a diagnosis or even a known category of disease. The approach that we have selected demands that you formulate a broad differential diagnosis; the position of the case in the book offers no clues. The child with a stiff neck may be suffering from meningitis, a brain tumor, cervical adenitis, a fractured vertebra, or an overdose. You won't know ahead of time if the problem is infectious, neurologic, traumatic, or toxicologic, because we didn't divide the cases into chapters or sections. After all, when you practice medicine, particularly in the emergency department or in an office setting with acutely ill children, you face the same dilemma of formulating a differential diagnosis without even knowing if you are in the right ballpark.

Having chosen a design that mimics clinical practice rather than a table of contents, we have taken care to make certain that our readers are not left feeling rudderless or thinking that we are simply lazy. Furthermore, we suspect that some readers will return to this book to review specific areas, either to satisfy their own curiosity or to prepare for an examination. Thus, we have provided two guides. The penultimate section of the book organizes topics in a standard fashion, predominantly by system, and lists relevant cases under each heading; those cases that apply to more than one topic have multiple listings. Then, with a bow to tradition, we conclude with a index, which highlights major themes in bold, making access to any specific information relatively effortless. Therefore, on a second (or third) go round, one may choose to use the book like a standard study guide.

We are already collecting more items for a second edition. Unlike most textbooks, every single image will need to be new, so we have our work cut out for us. We think you will enjoy *Pictorial Review of Pediatrics* and look forward to receiving any suggestions that you might put forth for our next volume.

Gary L. Fleisher
Stephen Ludwig

CONTENTS

CASE 1

This 3-year-old girl comes to the emergency department during the early autumn in Boston with a complaint of an earache. Her mother reports that the girl has been pulling at her ear and grimacing with pain. The child has been completely healthy previously with no prior ear infections. The current episode began gradually 24 hours ago and has not been accompanied by fever.

1. The most likely diagnosis is:
   A. Dental abscess
   B. Otitis media
   C. Temporomandibular joint arthritis
   D. Torticollis
   E. None of the above

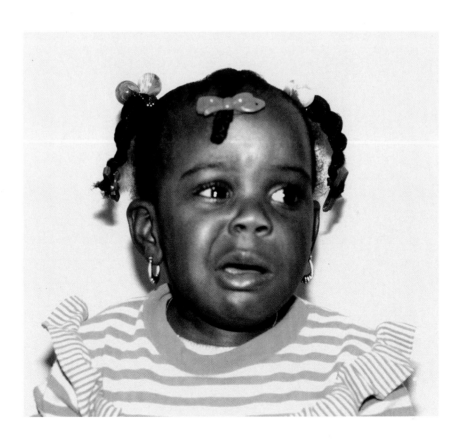

As you approach the patient to examine her ears, she begins to cry. Her head and neck are completely normal, including mobile, gray tympanic membranes bilaterally. Other than the observations in the photograph, further examination is non-revealing.

2. Which diagnostic study would you order?
   A. CT scan of the head
   B. Lumbar puncture
   C. Lyme titer
   D. Dental consult
   E. Sinus X-ray

3. Assume that the result of the diagnostic study is normal. Which drug is most likely to be useful for treatment?
   A. Prednisone orally
   B. Phenytoin orally
   C. Ampicillin orally
   D. Neomycin-hydrocortisone ear drops
   E. Ketorolac orally

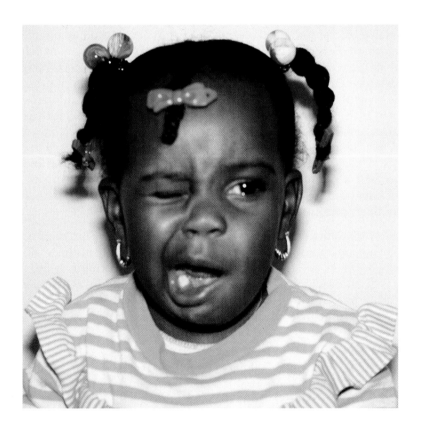

DISCUSSION

ANSWERS:
1. B. Otitis media
2. C. Lyme titer
3. A. Prednisone orally

1. At the time the question is posed, prior to obtaining further history or performing a physical examination, the most likely diagnosis is otitis media. Additional conditions in the differential diagnosis of ear pain include otitis externa, furuncle of the auditory canal, herpes zoster oticus, foreign body, traumatic lesions of the ear, dental abscess, pharyngitis or peritonsillar abscess, sinusitis, parotitis, temporomandibular arthritis, and miscellaneous conditions in anatomically related structures. Since the answer lies in the ear for 99% of cases, this site is the logical place to start. Overall, otitis media is far and away the most frequent offender, even in patients without a fever. During the warm weather among children who have been swimming, otitis externa ranks second in frequency. If both the external canal and the tympanic membrane are normal, and not just obscured by abundant cerumen, then it is time to consider some of the less common disorders on the list. In retrospect, you may notice some mild asymmetry to the child's facial expression. Although I wouldn't expect anyone to notice this on first inspection, give yourself credit if you chose "None of the above," based on your keen powers of observation.

2. The appropriate diagnostic test is a Lyme titer, as the child has Bell's palsy which is an isolated paralysis of the peripheral seventh nerve. Physical examination serves to rule out involvement of the central nucleus of the facial nerve (as patients with Bell's palsy cannot wrinkle their foreheads) or any other neurologic abnormality. A CT scan of the head is not indicated except in occasional cases when the neurologic examination is equivocal. Most cases of Bell's palsy are idiopathic. The most notable exception is Lyme disease, which may be responsible for over 50% of cases in endemic areas, such as the beaches and woods both north and south of Boston. While autumn is a bit late in the year for *Ixodes damini*, remember that the incubation period may be weeks, making an exposure over Labor Day a possibility. A lumbar puncture is indicated neither in idiopathic Bell's palsy nor with seventh cranial nerve paralysis secondary to Lyme disease. Unless evidence of a dental abscess or sinus infection is found, an evaluation for these conditions is not routinely performed in a child with Bell's palsy.

3. Although some authorities would disagree, the best answer is prednisone. Ampicillin would be a good choice for Lyme disease, but the serology in this child is negative. Similarly, a topical anti-infective/anti-inflammatory medication helps only if otitis externa is diagnosed. Since Bell's palsy is, at most, only mildly and transiently painful in the acute phase, a nonsteroidal anti-inflammatory agent, such as ibuprofen, is unnecessary. Phenytoin and other anticonvulsants are not indicated.

Further Discussion

Bell's palsy is an idiopathic, unilateral paralysis of the seventh cranial nerve due to edema in the portion of the nerve that passes through the facial canal within the temporal bone. In cases of facial palsy with an identified cause, otitis media is the most likely finding. Follow-up of all patients is important because the weakness does not resolve fully in some children. In addition to steroids, treatment includes attention to the eye on the affected side, which may become dry due to the loss of the ability to close the lid. A wetting agent should be described to provide prophylaxis against corneal injury.

CASE 2

A 4-year-old girl comes to the emergency department at noon with fever. Although in her usual state of good health the previous day, she awoke with a fever of 39.8°C at 7:15 AM. Her father reports that she has become increasingly restless during the course of the morning. On first glance, she is breathing noisily and in acute distress. You administer oxygen via face mask immediately.

1. While obtaining further history, you decide to:
   A. Insert an intravenous catheter
   B. Draw a blood gas
   C. Perform a Heimlich maneuver
   D. Administer intramuscular ceftriaxone
   E. None of the above

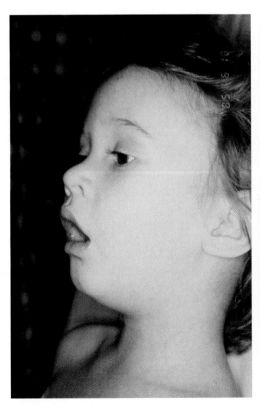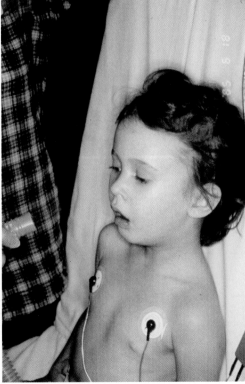

Further history indicates that she complained of a sore throat in the morning. She has not had a cough, vomiting, or diarrhea. The family moved to the United States three weeks ago from Central America. Vital signs include: T 39.4°C; P 128/min; R 32/min; BP 114/72 mm Hg. An X-ray is obtained.

2. Your diagnosis is:
   A. Epiglottitis
   B. Viral croup
   C. Spasmodic croup
   D. Retropharyngeal abscess
   E. Peritonsillar abscess

3. The preferred treatment for this disorder is:
   A. Tracheostomy
   B. Endotracheal intubation
   C. Nebulized racemic epinephrine
   D. Incision and drainage
   E. Intravenous clindamycin

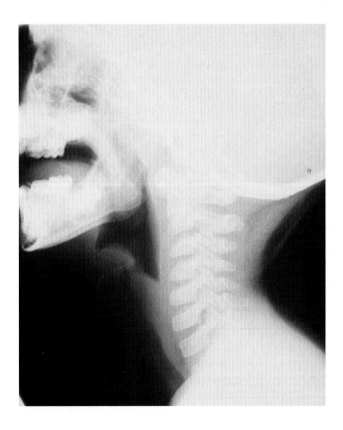

DISCUSSION

ANSWERS:
1. E. None of the above
2. A. Epiglottitis
3. B. Endotracheal Intubation

1. The correct answer is none of the above. A child with the sudden onset of respiratory distress, noisy breathing, and an anxious state most likely has an upper respiratory obstruction. Any painful procedure (insertion of an intravenous catheter, drawing an arterial blood gas, or giving an injection) risks agitating the child and converting a partial obstruction to a complete airway obstruction. In a 4-year-old with fever, who is moving air and has no specific history of a choking episode, the possibility of a foreign body is so remote that it precludes the use of the Heimlich maneuver prior to further diagnostic study. Reasonable steps would include either obtaining a portable lateral neck X-ray or inserting an endotracheal tube (most frequently in the operating room), depending on the adequacy of breathing and the skill of the physicians.

2. The most likely diagnosis is epiglottitis, given the uncertainty of immunization status, the age, the rapidity of onset, the height of the fever, and the appearance of the child. Viral croup usually occurs more often in children under the age of three years, has a gradual onset, and causes a low-grade fever. Spasmodic croup characteristically begins abruptly in the middle of the night. Peritonsillar abscess complicates a pre-existing pharyngitis and, thus, has a gradual onset. While characteristically causing a "hot potato" voice, being unilateral, peritonsillar abscess rarely leads to complete obstruction and air hunger. Retropharyngeal abscess is a good second choice, but the brief duration of symptoms weighs against this diagnosis.

3. The preferred treatment is endotracheal intubation, followed by intravenous antibiotics and intensive care. Tracheostomy is acceptable but more difficult to perform and is frequently accompanied by an increase in complications. Neither nebulized racemic epinephrine nor incision and drainage have a role, and clindamycin is not an appropriate antibiotic.

Further Discussion

Epiglottitis refers to inflammation of the epiglottis and surrounding structures, most often due to bacterial infection. Traditionally, *Hemophilus influenzae* has been the pathogen most often causing this disorder. However, disease from this organism is now rare among children who have received the conjugate vaccine. Other bacterial pathogens, such as Group A *Streptococcus*, or physical insults, such as thermal injury, are also considerations. The immediate concern in a child with epiglottitis is complete airway obstruction. If the diagnosis is strongly suspected or the child is not oxygenating adequately, the physician must rapidly secure the airway. In less pressing cases, a lateral neck X-ray, with appropriate attendance to the patient and preparation for management of the airway, should be obtained to assist in making a more specific diagnosis. Give a third-generation cephalosporin, such as cefotaxime or ceftriaxone, to cover the likely pathogens.

CASE 3

A 2-year-old girl was reaching into a sink filled with soapy water when she sustained the following injury on a broken glass. As you approach her, she withdraws and begins to shriek. Your best efforts to calm her down fail, not surprisingly, to gain even the slightest degree of cooperation.

1. You should:
   A. Sedate her and explore the wound
   B. Consult a surgeon
   C. Repair the wound under local anesthesia
   D. Persist in your attempts to gain cooperation
   E. Use the response to pinprick for evaluation

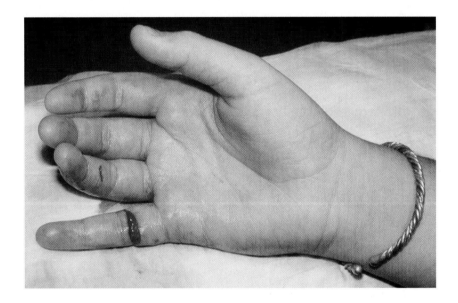

DISCUSSION

ANSWER:

1. **B. Consult a surgeon**

1. It makes little sense to do anything except call an appropriate surgeon, as merely looking at this child's hand from across the room shows that she has lacerated a flexor tendon. Patients at this age are unlikely to cooperate for a detailed neurovascular examination. While a careful exploration is certainly appropriate, lacerated flexor tendons notoriously retract and may not be seen; surgical consultation is indicated regardless of further findings. Pricking the distal portion of the child's finger with a pin will abolish any likelihood of establishing rapport with the patient and will most likely cause her to withdraw the entire hand rather than flex the finger.

Further Discussion

Two tendons control flexion of the fingers. The flexor digitorum profundus inserts on the distal phalanx and the flexor digitorum superficialis on the middle phalanx. Given the location of this wound, the superficialis has definitely been lacerated and the profundus may be involved as well. The most useful information in this case, as in many similar situations, is gleaned from observation of the child from afar before singling out the involved area. When evaluating a cooperative patient, flexion at both the distal interphalangeal and the proximal interphalangeal joints should be tested individually. Patients with partial tendon lacerations may display normal motor function. In these cases, careful exploration, which is always indicated, becomes paramount. If necessary, the child should be sedated. Achieving anesthesia with a digital block, rather than local infiltration, and the use of a tourniquet facilitate the identification of injuries to deeper structures. Magnifying loupes further enhance visualization.

Repair of flexor tendons generally requires use of the operating suite. The lacerated ends of the tendon retract and are not easily located and anastomosed. Many surgeons will perform the repair at the time of injury. However, it is equally acceptable in consultation to close the laceration to the skin and defer the definitive surgery. By way of contrast, extensor tendons are usually repaired in the emergency department.

A 9-month-old infant comes to the emergency department with rash involving most of his body. The first lesions appeared seven days earlier on his proximal right forearm and right antecubital fossa. According to his mother, his physician prescribed mupirocin. The rash spread despite therapy, and two days ago a second physician gave him erythromycin orally. Today, his mother became concerned because the lesions continued to extend over the entire body and the child seemed ill.

1. You recommend the following treatment:
   A. Acyclovir
   B. Silver sulfadiazine
   C. Prednisone
   D. Ceftriaxone
   E. Amphotericin

2. If not treated promptly, the likely outcome is:
   A. Severe scarring
   B. Death
   C. Pneumonia
   D. Renal failure
   E. Resolution

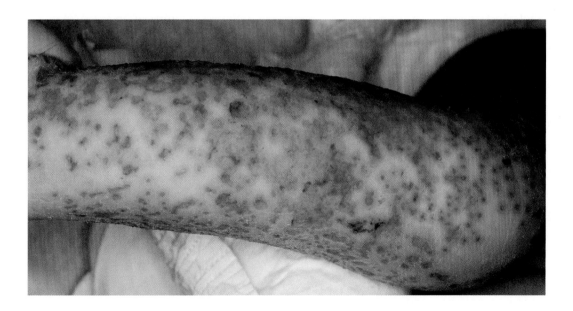

DISCUSSION

ANSWERS:

1. A. Acyclovir
2. B. Death

1. This boy has eczema herpeticum, a secondary infection by Herpes simplex virus of the eczematous lesions of atopic dermatitis. The recommended treatment is acyclovir, given intravenously when the lesions are extensive. In very localized cases, oral acyclovir suffices. Antibiotics, such as ceftriaxone, are indicated for bacterial superinfections in atopic dermatitis. While secondary bacterial infections outnumber cases of eczema herpeticum by several orders of magnitude, a few clues in this child point to the correct diagnosis of a viral process. Most importantly, ulcerated lesions, as seen here, are virtually pathognomonic of herpes. The absence of both impetiginized areas (crusted and oozing) and progression after several days of treatment with antibiotic agents sway one away from the diagnosis of a bacterial superinfection. Silver sulfadiazine, a popular therapy for burned patients, has no proven role in eczema herpeticum; amphotericin is an antifungal agent; and steroids are contraindicated.

2. Untreated, eczema herpeticum in this boy would most likely be fatal. Death results most frequently from the cutaneous involvement rather than systemic spread and visceral involvement, which are seen in neonates. Potential complications are similar to those observed in patients with major burns, including fluid and electrolyte disturbances and sepsis.

Further Discussion

Eczema herpeticum and eczema vaccinatum are viral infections with a similar appearance that affect patients with atopic dermatitis. Subsequent to the discontinuation of vaccination against smallpox, eczema vaccinatum no longer occurs. This child exhibits the characteristic lesions of eczema herpeticum, punched out ulcers. In general, herpetic infections of the skin are characterized by vesicles. Although vesicles may be seen in patients with eczema herpeticum, more often than not, they are absent. I hypothesize that the severe pruritus that accompanies both atopic dermatitis and herpes leads to the rapid obliteration of vesicles and facilitates the evolution of ulcers.

When patients with known atopic dermatitis seek treatment for flare ups of their disease, three explanations are possible: bacterial superinfection, viral superinfection, or simple worsening of the basic process. Differentiation between these three causes is important because the treatments (antibiotic agents, antiviral therapy, and corticosteroids) are quite different. In my experience, Herpes simplex is the explanation that is most frequently overlooked.

A 7-year-old boy arrives in the emergency department by ambulance. The paramedics report that they were summoned to the house for a child with seizures. Upon their arrival, they found the child as pictured below. They were unable to establish intravenous access and transported him to your hospital, as a priority one run. An accompanying adult, the boyfriend of the child's mother, states that he is not aware of any history of seizures. He does note that the boy has been taking two teaspoons (320 mg) of acetaminophen every four hours over the last two days for a "cold." On arrival his vital signs are as follows: P 110/min; R 24/min; BP 125/85 mm Hg; T 37.8°C.

1. You order the following diagnostic study:
   A. Lumbar puncture
   B. X-ray of the neck
   C. CT scan of head
   D. Neurologic consultation
   E. Toxicology screen

2. You treat with:
   A. Naloxone
   B. Phenytoin
   C. Lorazepam
   D. Diphenhydramine
   E. Thiopental/succinylcholine

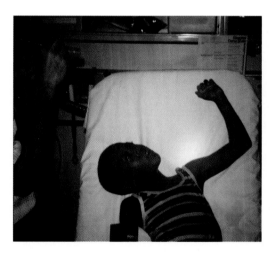
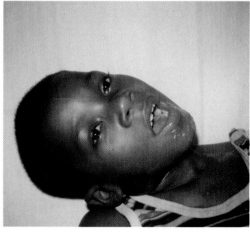

You have treated the child with intravenous medication and he appears as shown 30 seconds afterwards. Subsequently, the result of the diagnostic study that you obtained returns as normal. The boy's mother arrives, and on further questioning denies prior seizures, any recent trauma, or the presence of any prescription drugs in the house.

3. Your diagnosis is:
   A. Tonic clonic seizure
   B. Epilepsia partialis continua
   C. Dystonic reaction
   D. Torticollis
   E. Retropharyngeal abscess

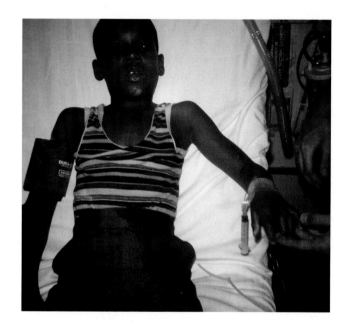

DISCUSSION

ANSWERS:
1. E. Toxicology screen
2. D. Diphenhydramine
3. C. Dystonic reaction

1. The diagnostic study of choice is a toxicology screen, as the child is having a dystonic reaction. Cerebellar tumors are a rare cause of abnormal posturing and would be diagnosed with imaging, using either CT or, better yet, MR scanning. If you suspected torticollis (particularly with a history of preceding trauma) or a retropharyngeal abscess, then you might reasonably order a cervical spine series or soft tissue X-rays of the neck. The story of an acute, perhaps febrile, illness, being treated with acetaminophen, raises the specter of meningitis, which is diagnosed by lumbar puncture. However, the boy is afebrile (virtually unheard of with symptomatic bacterial meningitis beyond the first month or two of life) and holds his head cocked to one side, which is not indicative of nuchal rigidity. If you made a diagnosis of a focal seizure from these still photographs, I could not fault you. On the other hand, I see no purpose for a neurologic consultation.

2. The treatment of choice for this boy is intravenous diphenhydramine. Naloxone would be indicated for an overdose of narcotics, usually manifest as somnolence or coma, and either phenytoin (soon to be replaced by fosphenytoin) or lorazepam are excellent choices for the initial management of generalized tonic-clonic seizures. Except in the face of respiratory compromise, rapid induction of anesthesia with thiopental and succinylcholine followed by endotracheal intubation would not be wise.

3. As expected, the patient responded rapidly to intravenous diphenhydramine with resolution of his dystonic reaction. Although caused by an ingestion, the toxicology screen may be negative. The reaction is idiosyncratic rather than dose related, and may occur 8-10 hours after an exposure; thus, trace levels of some substances may not be detected. In this case, once the child recovered, he revealed that he had ingested a pill that he found on the living room floor of his home. While the family did not keep any prescription drugs in the house, a visiting maternal grandmother later remembered that she had dropped her haloperidol from her purse.

Further Discussion

Phenothiazines and butyrophenones, which are the most commonly prescribed major tranquilizers, cause the majority of dystonic reactions. This clinical syndrome is characterized by episodic spasm of voluntary muscles, particularly those of the head and neck. Additionally, patients may develop torticollis, tongue protrusion, or oculogyric crisis. Treatment with either diphenhydramine (Benadryl®) or benztropine (Cogentin®), intravenously, provides prompt relieve. A prescription for two days of oral therapy is indicated to prevent recurrences, as the offending agent may outlast the antidote in the bloodstream.

A 2-year-old boy has had a lesion on his parietal scalp just above his ear for 1 month. His mother used a special shampoo for two weeks, and then an ointment for 10 days, without improvement.

1. You recommend:
    A. Incision and drainage
    B. Clotrimazole cream
    C. Griseofulvin suspension
    D. Erythromycin suspension
    E. Prednisolone suspension

2. You advise her to return if the lesion has not resolved in:
    A. 3 days
    B. 1 week
    C. 2 weeks
    D. 4 weeks
    E. 8 weeks

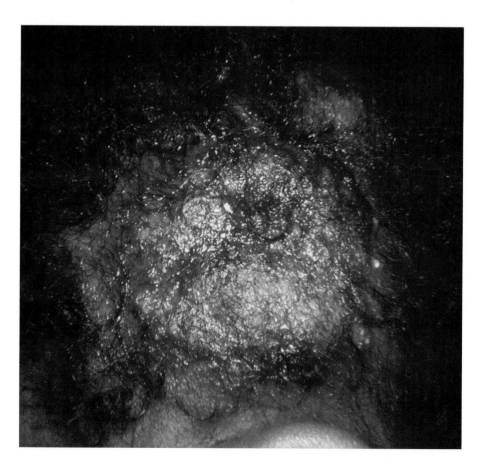

DISCUSSION

ANSWERS:

1. C. **Griseofulvin suspension**
2. E. **8 weeks**

1. This boy has a kerion, which is an inflammatory lesion that develops secondary to tinea capitis. The correct treatment is griseofulvin administered for a minimum of 6 weeks or until the lesion resolves. Other antifungal agents, such as ketoconazole, are effective, although there is less clinical experience with their use. Topical antifungal agents work remarkably well against tinea corporis but have no role in treating lesions that have even minimal involvement of the hair on the scalp or the eyebrows. While some authorities postulate that antibiotic and anti-inflammatory agents, such as erythromycin and prednisolone, may hasten the resolution of a kerion, this remains unproven. Certainly when used alone, these drugs have no effect. Incision and drainage is contraindicated, as surgical therapy provides no benefit, and the inflamed tissues heal slowly.

2. A kerion will rarely resolve in less than 6 weeks. I advise patients to return if a discernable decrease in the lesion size is not noted by 3 weeks and to return for a re-evaluation and a refill of the prescription for griseofulvin at 6–8 weeks if the lesion has not resolved. Although some authors recommend baseline and then periodic measurements of hepatic enzymes due to the risk of liver toxicity from griseofulvin, this complication is quite rare and makes routine chemical surveillance unnecessary in my opinion.

Further Discussion

A kerion arises after infection with dermatophytid fungi from one of three species: *Trichophyton*, *Microsporum*, or *Epidermophyton*. Several decades ago, the most common agent was *M. audouini*, which fluoresces under ultraviolet light. More recently, *T. tonsurans* has taken over and this organism does not fluoresce. Generally, the absolutely characteristic appearance of a kerion suffices to make the diagnosis. The lesion is boggy, exudative, greasy, and covered with thin, matted hair. If one is uncertain about the nature of the lesion, a culture provides definitive proof of the etiology. A specimen for culture is obtained by scraping the lesion or rubbing it with a sterile toothbrush and placing the collected material on Sabouraud dextrose agar; growth of the organism requires 1 to 3 weeks. Treatment may be initiated with griseofulvin while awaiting the results of culture or withheld until a report has returned. Selenium sulfide shampoo reduces spore counts and provides adjunctive therapy.

CASE 7

An 18-year-old woman complains of shortness of breath. Six days earlier, she developed high spiking fevers and was placed on amoxicillin. Four days ago, she developed a rash. Her physician discontinued amoxicillin. The rash, which began on her chest and neck, has now spread to involve most of her body. Oximetry shows a saturation of 80% on room air. You initiate oxygen therapy and obtain an X-ray of the chest.

1. You anticipate that the chest X-ray shows:
   A. An interstitial infiltrate
   B. Massive cardiomegaly
   C. A large pleural effusion
   D. Widening of the mediastinum
   E. A lobar infiltrate

2. Breathing 100% oxygen, her saturation increases to 96%. You initiate therapy with:
   A. Erythromycin
   B. Acyclovir
   C. Thoracentesis
   D. Ciprofloxacin
   E. Mediastinal radiation

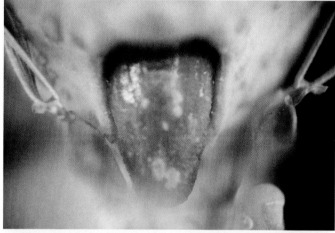

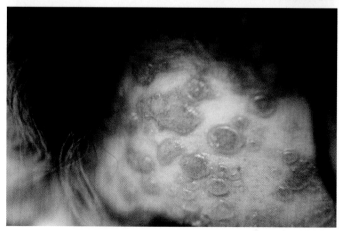

DISCUSSION

ANSWERS:
1. **A. Interstitial infiltrate**
2. **B. Acyclovir**

1. The chest X-ray will show a diffuse, "millet seed," interstitial infiltrate characteristic of varicella pneumonia. Other causes of shortness of breath with fever include bacterial pneumonia (lobar infiltrate and/or pleural effusion on X-ray), myocarditis (cardiomegaly), viral or bacterial pericarditis (pericardial effusion), and lymphoma causing superior vena cava syndrome (widened mediastinum). None of these entities would cause the diffuse vesiculobullous exanthem and enanthem exhibited by this patient.

2. The treatment of choice for varicella with severe pneumonia is intravenous acyclovir. Erythromycin would be indicated for atypical pneumonias (*Mycoplasma*, *Legionella*). Ciprofloxacin is a reasonable choice, but not a common one, for a young adult with a community-acquired bacterial infection of the lungs. If a large pleural effusion is detected in a febrile patient with respiratory distress, thoracentesis may be both diagnostic and therapeutic. In children with superior vena cava syndrome from mediastinal lymphoma, immediate radiation therapy, prior to establishing a tissue diagnosis, is the treatment of choice.

Further Discussion

Varicella is a ubiquitous infection of childhood. Although a decrease in the incidence will follow the widespread usage of the vaccine in the future, the rate of infection remains high. Most cases affect preschool and school age children. Those few individuals who escape childhood infection risk severe disease in adulthood. As seen in this case, the cutaneous and mucosal lesions are more extensive than normally seen in immunocompetent children, with nearly confluent bullae replacing the typical isolated vesicles and pustules. Approximately 5% of young adults with varicella develop radiographic evidence of pneumonia which is frequently severe. Varicella causes a diffuse pulmonary infection with a characteristic "millet seed" appearance. When instituted early in the course, treatment with acyclovir effectively contains the infection. I routinely prescribe acyclovir to all patients with varicella under 6 months or over 15 years of age, as these groups tend to have the most pronounced manifestations.

This 14-old boy complains of pain in his left shoulder.

1. Your diagnosis is:
   A. Septic arthritis of the shoulder
   B. Dislocation of the shoulder
   C. Fracture of the clavicle
   D. Separation of the shoulder
   E. Displaced Salter I fracture of the humerus

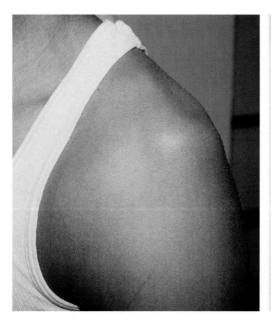 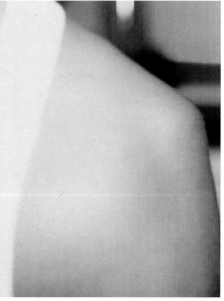

You obtain an X-ray.

2. To treat this problem, you:
   A. Administer antibiotics
   B. Apply traction-countertraction
   C. Place a clavicle strap
   D. Recommend operative repair
   E. Use a sling and swathe

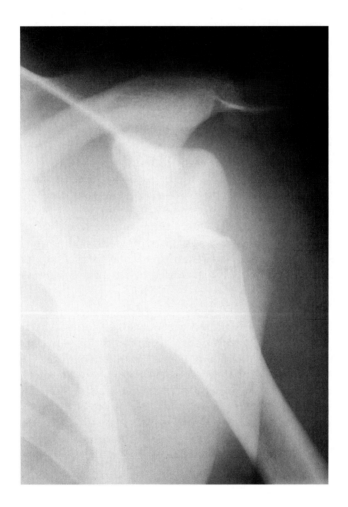

DISCUSSION

ANSWERS:
1. **B. Dislocation of the shoulder**
2. **B. Apply traction-countertraction**

1. The shoulder is foreshortened and has lost its normal convex contour, revealing instead the concavity of the glenoid fossa. Thus, the patient has sustained a dislocation of the shoulder. Septic arthritis in the shoulder, which is surrounded by thick musculature in adolescence, generally produces no change in the outward appearance of the joint, although the patient will complain of severe pain with movement. With a fracture of the clavicle, some shortening may be noticeable, but the contour of the shoulder is unchanged. A shoulder separation causes tenderness over the acromioclavicular ligament and widening of the acromioclavicular joint on X-ray, particularly when obtained with the patient holding weights. A Salter I fracture of the humerus would manifest itself with swelling, point tenderness, and, in some cases, deformity of the proximal portion of the arm.

2. The X-ray shows a dislocation of the shoulder, as the humeral head lies inferior to the glenoid fossa. In this particular boy, the humeral head dislocated anteriorly (this occurs in 90% of cases), but a scapular or Y view is needed to determine the direction of displacement radiographically. Many techniques are available for relocation of the humeral head, of which the application of traction-countertraction is one of the more widely practiced. The clavicle is not seen to be fractured, so a clavicle strap (which has replaced the traditional "figure-of-eight" dressing) is not indicated. Similarly, a humeral fracture, usually treated with a sling and swathe or a shoulder immobilizer, is not present. Septic arthritis causes no radiographic abnormalities. As discussed above, X-rays of a patient with an acromioclavicular sprain (shoulder separation) may be abnormal only when the joint is stressed by having the patient hold weights.

Further Discussion

As with many other situations, children are not small adults when it comes to their shoulders. The same forces that cause separations and dislocations in teenagers produce physeal (Salter) fractures in prepubertal patients. This difference exists because the weakest point around the joint in young children is the physis, which will give way before the acromioclavicular ligament or the joint capsule tears. Regardless of the maneuver chosen for reduction, I find the use of muscle relaxants and analgesics to be helpful in muscular adolescent males. My combination of choice for the teenager is intravenous midazolam (2-4 mg) and fentanyl (100-250 µg), titrated to effect while monitoring the oxygen saturation. You will often need to apply slow, steady traction for several minutes and should not be discouraged by failure to reduce the dislocation immediately.

A 15-year-old girl complains of having chills and feeling stiff. Her temperature is 38.3°C. The only finding on examination is a scattered eruption of approximately 12 lesions, including the hands (web space) and feet (sole) as shown here.

1. The best diagnostic study is:
   A. Immunofluorescence of a lesion
   B. Culture of the blood
   C. Echocardiogram
   D. Culture of the cervix
   E. Aspiration of bone marrow

2. This disease does not occur in:
   A. Elementary school-age girls
   B. Males
   C. Patients over age 30 years
   D. Properly immunized individuals
   E. Inhabitants of cold climates

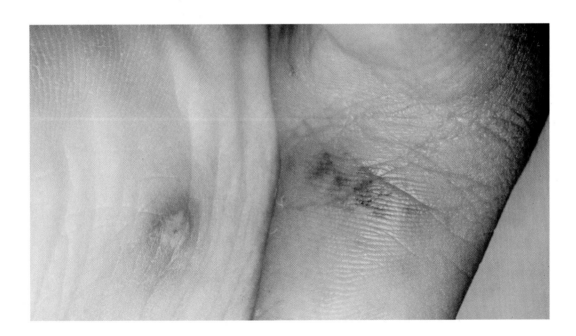

DISCUSSION

ANSWERS:
1. **D. Culture of the cervix**
2. **A. Elementary school-age girls**

1. The diagnosis is disseminated gonorrhea or gonococcemia, and the best test is a culture of the cervix. The symptoms and signs (multiple small joint arthralgias and cutaneous lesions) result from the deposition of antigen-antibody complexes. Thus, blood cultures will be negative. If one suspected either Herpes simplex or varicella-zoster virus infection, immunofluorescent staining of a scraping from the lesions is a very sensitive diagnostic technique. Septic emboli seen in patients with subacute bacterial endocarditis or leukemia with sepsis, particularly with *Pseudomonas aeruginosa*, have a very similar appearance. If not previously diagnosed, an echocardiogram to detect valvular lesions in the heart or aspiration of bone marrow looking for evidence of neoplastic infiltration would be helpful to make these diagnoses. Given the brief history and the absence of suggestive physical findings for either subacute endocarditis (murmur, Osler's nodes, Janeway lesions) or leukemia (pallor, petechiae, splenomegaly), such illnesses are much less likely than gonorrhea, which is epidemic among teenagers.

2. Disseminated gonorrhea does not occur among elementary school-age girls. The organism establishes an infection in the endocervix of postpubertal females and ascends during menses. In prepubertal girls, gonorrhea may produce a vaginitis, as the unestrogenized epithelium is susceptible to infection, but neither cause cervicitis nor ascends further. Gonorrhea affects sexually active males and females of all ages in all climates. It causes approximately one million infections annually in the United States and is second in frequency only to *Chlamydia trachomatis*. While the incidence is highest during late adolescence and into the third decade, sexually active individuals over 30 years old may contract disseminated gonorrhea.

Further Discussion

The most common manifestation of disseminated gonococcemia is the arthritis-dermatitis syndrome, which begins with additive polyarthralgias, usually involving the knees and the small joints of the hands. After a few days, characteristic skin lesions, as shown here, appear in 75% of patients. Untreated, potential complications include frank septic arthritis, and, less commonly, endocarditis, meningitis, and overwhelming sepsis. Most commonly, the initial therapy is intravenous ceftriaxone.

The father of this 7-month-old boy seeks care for his son for a swollen scrotum. The child is otherwise healthy and has no additional symptoms.

1. The therapy you recommend is:
   A. Immediate detorsion
   B. Delayed herniorrhaphy
   C. Observation
   D. Trimethoprim sulfamethoxazole
   E. None of the above

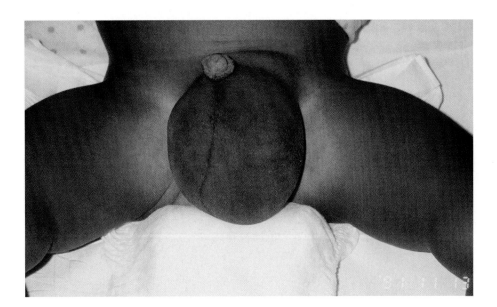

DISCUSSION

ANSWER:

1. B. Delayed herniorrhaphy

1. The correct answer is delayed herniorrhaphy. The differential diagnosis includes torsion of the testis, torsion of the appendix testis, testicular hydrocele, inguinal hernia, and epididymitis/orchitis. Additionally, one needs to determine if an inguinal hernia is reducible, incarcerated (irreducible), or strangulated (incarcerated and with ischemic tissue). An irreducible hernia or one that is strangulated requires immediate surgery. In this case, both the degree of swelling and the presence of a bulge in the inguinal area point to a hernia as the diagnosis. Generally, large hernias, such as this, are easily reducible. In addition, the absence of symptoms (irritability, vomiting) and signs (abdominal distention) weigh against incarceration or strangulation. Testicular hydroceles usually appear earlier in infancy and do not reach this size. Similarly, the testicular swelling with testicular torsion, and also with torsion of an appendix testis, is neither this marked nor asymptomatic. The scrotum may appear generally discolored with testicular torsion or an isolated blue dot may be seen overlying a twisted appendix.

Further Discussion

Indirect inguinal hernia is the most common congenital anomaly in children, affecting males 10 times more frequently than females. Incarceration may occur at any age; when encountered, immediate reduction should be attempted. This is facilitated in all cases by placing the child in a Trendelenburg position. Until reduction is achieved, oral intake should be stopped. The technique for reduction calls for placement of one hand over the inguinal ring, forming a funnel for the contents of the hernia sac, while the other hand milks the gas or fluid out of the entrapped bowel back into the abdominal intestines, using circumferentially applied pressure. In rare cases sedation is required with an agent such as morphine, 0.1 mg/kg.

The father of a 4-year-old boy complains that his son has been refusing to drink fluids for 36 hours. The child's illness began 5 days ago with a fever that has persisted and climbed as high as 39.5°C. This morning the child seemed lethargic to his parents. On examination, his vital signs are: T 39.3°C; P 130/min: R 30 min; BP 95/55 mm Hg. His mucous membranes are dry but not parched, and his skin turgor is decreased without tenting. The remainder of the exam is normal except as shown:

1. The most effective treatment for this problem is:
   A. Oral acyclovir
   B. Intravenous acyclovir
   C. Topical xylocaine
   D. Oral clindamycin
   E. Topical nystatin

2. This condition is most commonly seen in:
   A. Newborns
   B. Preschoolers
   C. Adolescents
   D. Young adults
   E. Older adults

3. Managed with the treatment recommended by you in question #1, the disease will resolve in:
   A. 1 to 2 days
   B. 4 to 5 days
   C. 8 to 10 days
   D. 3 to 4 weeks
   E. 2 to 3 months

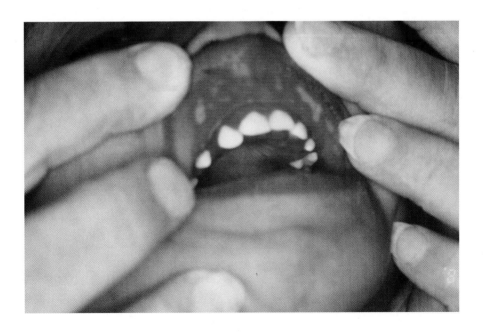

DISCUSSION

ANSWERS:
1. B. Topical xylocaine
2. B. Preschoolers
3. C. 8 to 10 days

1. The only potentially correct answer is viscous xylocaine which provides a modicum of topical anesthesia for patients with primary herpetic stomatitis as shown here. Studies have found that use of acyclovir does not shorten the course of primary herpetic stomatitis in immunocompetent children with otherwise uncomplicated infections. Antibiotics play no role in herpetic infections. A disease that may sometimes be confused with herpetic stomatitis is acute necrotizing ulcerative gingivostomatitis (ANUG), which is an invasion of the gums by anaerobic bacteria. For this infection, clindamycin provides excellent therapy. Monilia causes whitish plaques, usually on the tongue and buccal mucosa, and responds favorably to oral nystatin.

2. Primary herpetic stomatitis may occur at any age but most commonly affects preschoolers. The prevalence of antibodies to Herpes simplex virus rises most rapidly in populations of lower socioeconomic status, as crowding living quarters facilitate the spread of the virus. Thus, among patients from more affluent backgrounds, primary infections occur frequently in later childhood and adolescence. Recurrent infections ("cold sores") similarly affect patients of all ages, but are more common in teenagers than in preschoolers. Extensive involvement during a recurrence is unusual except among immunosuppressed patients.

3. Given that antiviral therapy does not abbreviate the duration of the lesions, it is unfortunate that primary herpetic stomatitis, while self-limited in the immunocompetent host, lasts in most cases for 8-12 days.

Further Discussion

Children with primary herpetic gingivostomatitis are often quite miserable and may refuse to accept oral intake. The majority will respond to prolonged, gentle coaxing. Cool liquids, such as juices or popsicles, may soothe the lesions. Avoid orange or lemon juices which contain citric acid. When oral hydration proves impossible, intravenous fluids may be necessary. Often a bolus of normal saline, at 20 cc/kg, followed by 5% dextrose/0.5% normal saline for several hours in the emergency department will be sufficient.

CASE 12

The 4-year-old girl arrives by ambulance. As she hits the stretcher, one of the paramedics reports that she is a known "epileptic," under treatment with phenobarbital for the past 6 months, who began to convulse approximately 15 minutes ago. They maintained her on 100% oxygen by mask during the transport but have been unable to establish intravenous (IV) access. On first glance, she appears acutely ill with a poor respiratory effort and tonic-clonic seizure activity. The monitor displays a pattern captured moments later on the tracing below.

1. As the initial step, you:
   A. Insert an endotracheal tube
   B. Place a peripheral IV
   C. Obtain a 12-lead EKG
   D. Defibrillate
   E. None of the above

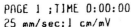

PAGE 1 ; TIME 0:00:00
25 mm/sec; 1 cm/mV

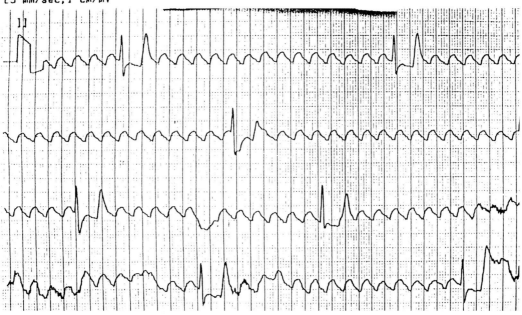

2. You and the "IV nurse" have been unsuccessful in establishing peripheral intravenous access after 3 minutes. A respiratory therapist is providing manual ventilation, and the patient's oxygen saturation is 95%. Although she improved with some of your initial maneuvers, she continues to convulse. The tracing on the monitor is the same as upon her arrival. One of the paramedics is attempting to insert an intraosseous needle. You decide to:
   A. Place a catheter percutaneously in the femoral vein
   B. Place a catheter percutaneously in the internal jugular vein
   C. Place a catheter percutaneously in the subclavian vein
   D. Perform a cutdown on the greater saphenous vein
   E. Continue to attempt peripheral venous cannulation

DISCUSSION

ANSWERS:

1. E. None of the above
2. A. Place a catheter percutaneously in the femoral vein

1. The rhythm shows atrial flutter with characteristic "saw-tooth" waves and occasional narrow-complex ventricular activity. Since the treatment of choice is synchronous cardioversion, none of the answers is correct. One might argue for endotracheal intubation, given the presence of poor respiratory effort. However, I suspect it would be difficult to intubate this patient while she is having tonic-clonic activity without using a muscle relaxant, which is best delivered intravenously. Most patients have a poor respiratory effort during a generalized seizure, but can be adequately oxygenated. Additionally, cardioversion can be performed in 5 to 10 seconds and offers an opportunity to instantly remedy the arrhythmia, and perhaps the entire problem. Both IV access and a 12-lead EKG will be essential, but neither takes priority over cardioversion and management of the airway.

2. My choice is percutaneous catheterization of the femoral vein. On the other hand, I'll give full credit for any answer, except continued attempts to achieve peripheral access. This situation deserves a more aggressive approach. If one is skilled at cannulation of the internal jugular or subclavian veins, both routes are acceptable. However, I would anticipate encountering difficulties in this small child who is actively convulsing and receiving manual ventilation. The physical constraints may make it hard to access and properly position her neck, and the risk of pneumothorax while attempting to catheterize the subclavian vein of a moving target concerns me. I know that a cutdown of the greater saphenous would occupy me for at least 5 to 10 minutes, a good deal longer than would using the Seldinger technique to access the femoral vein, so this technique would not be my first choice.

Further Discussion

This girl had a cardiomyopathy. In retrospect, her prior seizures were secondary to short runs of atrial flutter, leading to hypoxia. On previous occasions, the arrhythmia had resolved by the time she reached a medical facility and escaped detection. Review of an electroencephalogram (EEG) obtained 1 week after her first seizure showed evidence of a conduction disturbance on the single electrocardiographic lead displayed at the bottom of the EEG tracing.

Atrial flutter is an arrhythmia that occurs infrequently in childhood. The treatment of choice is synchronous cardioversion, starting at 0.25 J/kg. If the patient does not respond, the dose of electricity should be doubled.

This 14-year-old female comes to the emergency department with increasing abdominal pain over the last few days. Today she had difficulty urinating. She has had no vomiting or diarrhea and is unclear as to how long the pain has been present. She denies dysuria, urinary frequency, fever, and is premenarchial. Her lower abdomen is diffusely tender. When you examine her abdomen and external genitalia you see the following.

1. The patient may need the following procedure or test tonight:
   A. Laparoscopy
   B. Bladder catheterization
   C. Cervical cultures
   D. Chemotherapy
   E. Pregnancy test

2. After relief of her symptoms by the above procedure, she needs referral to a specialist for the following condition:
   A. Pregnancy
   B. Sarcoma botryoides
   C. Congenital anomaly
   D. Dysfunctional uterine bleeding
   E. Wilm's tumor

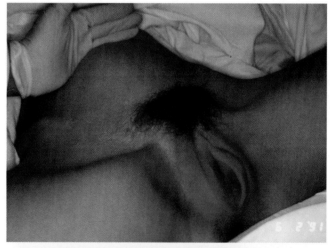

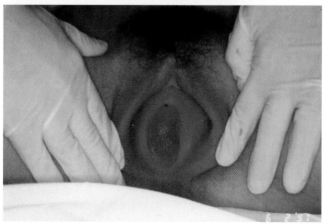

DISCUSSION

ANSWERS:

1. B. Bladder catheterization
2. C. Congenital anomaly

1. If the patient has urinary retention, she may require bladder catheterization. Her lower abdominal mass is a distended uterus and does not require laparoscopy. She has no findings suggestive of a sexually transmitted disease and does not need cervical cultures, nor does she require chemotherapy, since she does not have a tumor. Her primary amenorrhea is caused by blockage of menstrual blood due to her imperforate hymen.

2. Her external genital examination demonstrates Tanner IV pubic hair and a bulging bluish membrane over her vaginal introitus. The bluish color is caused by hematocolpos due to accumulating blood distending a congenitally imperforate hymen, as this young woman reaches menarche. In sarcoma botryoides, a "grape like" mass may protrude from the vagina. In dysfunctional uterine bleeding, Wilm's tumor or pregnancy, the patient may have lower abdominal pain, but should have normal external genitalia.

Further Discussion

This congenital vaginal obstruction is usually diagnosed during routine examinations or in infancy when mucous secretions distend the vagina and cause mucocolpos and urinary retention. If not noted then, the obstruction will remain dormant until puberty and then cause abdominal pain (sometimes cyclic), urinary symptoms (dysuria, urgency, or difficulty urinating), or primary amenorrhea. Once diagnosed, a gynecology consult should be obtained for surgical excision of the hymen within the next few days.

The parents of this 16-month-old seek care for fever and a red rash. Until 4 hours ago the child was well. On examination, his temperature is 39.4°C. and the rash is warm.

1. The most likely diagnosis is:
    A. Adenitis
    B. Fifth disease
    C. Buccal cellulitis
    D. Erysipelas
    E. Parotitis

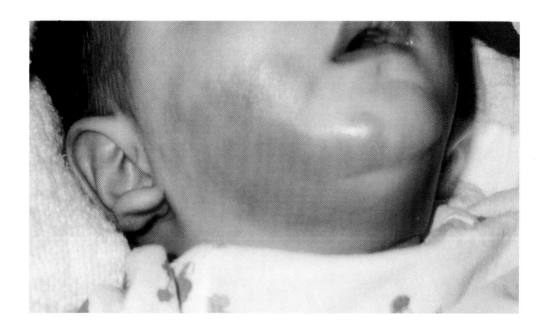

DISCUSSION

ANSWER:

1. D. Erysipelas

1. This child has a warm, red, sharply demarcated lesion consistent with erysipelas. An infected submandibular lymph node or salivary gland could look similar but would not usually be so well demarcated. A tender focal mass should be visible and palpable. Children with Fifth disease are usually afebrile and have bright red cheeks (the so-called "slapped cheek" appearance). The swelling of parotitis is over the angle of the jaw.

Further Discussion

Erysipelas is a superficial group A beta-hemolytic streptococcal infection. The skin is red, warm, tender, indurated, and has a sharply demarcated edge. If untreated, it may progress rapidly to bacteremia and necrotizing myositis or fasciitis. Management consists of antibiotic therapy with penicillin or a cephalosporin. Initially, a cephalosporin is preferred to provide coverage for the spectrum of pathogens that cause facial cellulitis. Once the specific diagnosis of erysipelas is made clinically or by culture, penicillin at 250,000 units/kg is the drug of choice.

A 2-year-old girl has had this red pruritic rash for 1 day. She has been well except for a "runny" nose and a low-grade fever for the last 3 days. Her mother administered a teaspoon of diphenhydramine without any effect today.

1. For immediate relief you give:
   A. Amoxicillin
   B. Prednisone
   C. Subcutaneous epinephrine (1:1000)
   D. Another teaspoon of diphenhydramine
   E. Hydroxyzine

2. The most likely cause of these lesions is:
   A. Parvovirus B19
   B. Herpes simplex virus
   C. Idiopathic
   D. Drug ingestion
   E. Cold exposure

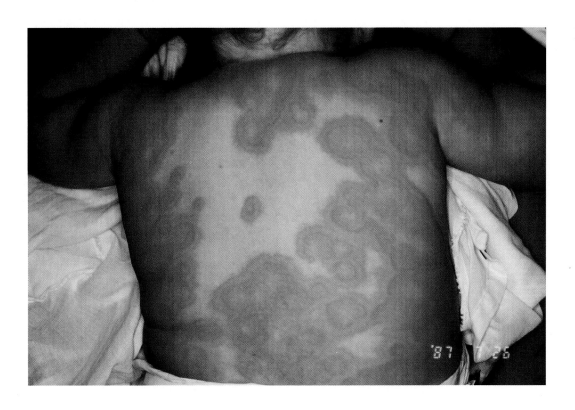

DISCUSSION

ANSWERS:
1. C. Subcutaneous epinephrine (1:1000)
2. C. Idiopathic

1. The rash is urticaria and the most rapid relief for the pruritus and resolution of the lesions is obtained with subcutaneous epinephrine (1:1000) at a dose of 0.01 cc/kg, maximum dose 0.3 cc. For more prolonged effects, I usually use Sus-phrin, the 1:200 aqueous suspension, at a dose of 0.05 cc/kg, maximum dose 0.15 cc.

2. In children, the cause of acute urticaria is rarely determined (i.e., idiopathic). The lesions are frequently associated with a preceding or concomitant viral infection. Drug exposure, foods, bites and stings are occasionally the cause. Urticaria are rarely caused by physical agents (heat, cold, or pressure), neoplasms, hepatitis B infection, or connective tissue diseases. Parvovirus B19 is associated with erythema infectiosum or Fifth disease which usually presents as facial erythema "slapped cheeks," progressing to a lacy macular rash on the extremities. Herpes simplex virus is associated with erythema multiforme.

Further Discussion

The child has acute onset of a pruritic rash that consists of large raised blanching wheals or hives. The skin is discolored but normal. Solid, raised, red, flat topped lesions are usually vascular reactions of some type, such as urticaria (in this case) or erythema multiforme. These two rashes are often confused. Urticaria are common, appear acutely, frequently change over a few hours, and although the central areas may be discolored, the skin is normal. Erythema multiforme are somewhat unusual, appear over a few days, stay in fixed locations, and the central areas may blister and crust. The "target lesion" of erythema multiforme has three zones, a central dusky, bullous or crusted area surrounded by a pale ring of edema and an outer red rim.

A 3-year-old boy, previously healthy except for a 2-day history of a upper respiratory infection, began complaining to his father about a sore throat after eating "chunky" chicken soup for lunch. His father measured his temperature at 101°F and had him lie down in his bed. When he checked on his son 3 hours later, he recorded a temperature of 102.5°F. The boy refused all liquids. The father was concerned that the boy's breathing seemed labored and brought him to the hospital.

At triage, the nurse notes mild stridor. She looks into his mouth and pages you to come to her area stat.

1. The cause of this boy's problem is:
   A. *Hemophilus influenzae*
   B. Thermal injury
   C. Parainfluenza virus
   D. A piece of chicken
   E. A congenital anomaly

2. Having made your diagnosis, you proceed to:
   A. Give oxygen
   B. Administer dexamethasone
   C. Perform endotracheal intubation
   D. Place a peripheral intravenous line
   E. Deliver four abdominal thrusts

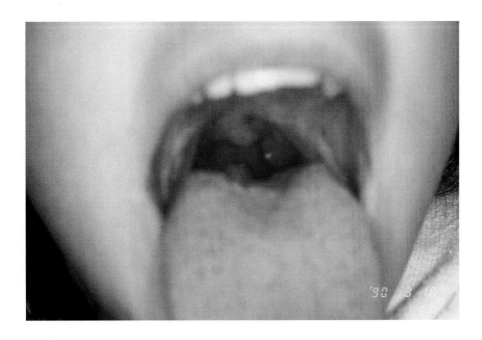

DISCUSSION

ANSWERS:
1. C. Parainfluenza virus
2. B. Administer dexamethasone

1. The nurse shows you a child with a normal pharynx and epiglottis. In a febrile 3-year-old with the onset of mild stridor that develops 2 days after the onset of a URI, the most likely diagnosis is croup, or viral laryngotracheobronchitis due to parainfluenza virus. He is at the upper end of the age range and his temperature is a tad higher than average, but neither of these findings is sufficient to detract from the diagnosis. Other entities to consider, particularly if you disregard the preceding URI, include bacterial and thermal (from the hot soup) epiglottitis and foreign body aspiration. With infection or burn injury to the epiglottis, it should appear red and inflamed. Additionally, one would presume the child has received immunizations against *Hemophilus influenzae* type b, virtually eliminating the possibility of an infection with this pathogen. Since the father offered no history of a choking episode during lunch nor did he describe a precipitous onset of stridor immediately after the child ate the "chunky" chicken soup, aspiration of a foreign body drops down on the list. While some patients develop a pneumonia behind an aspirated foreign body, fever would not be expect to occur for at least 12 to 24 hours.

2. The majority, but not unanimous, opinion holds that dexamethasone ameliorates the edema of the airway to some degree in viral croup. While oxygen would be harmless, patients with mild upper respiratory obstruction are not usually hypoxic. Endotracheal intubation by a skilled operator under controlled circumstances is the way to go with epiglottitis. Since nothing in the story calls for urgent intravenous therapy, it would seem reasonable to delay in this regard. Abdominal thrusts (Heimlich maneuver) are contraindicated. Even if you strongly suspect a foreign body, you should not perform abdominal thrusts on a child who is conscious and moving air adequately.

Further Discussion

The epiglottis comes into view at the base of the tongue during routine examination without instrumentation in 10 to 20% of children. In cases of epiglottitis, the swollen, red epiglottitis is potentially visualized even more frequently. Traditionally, the authorities tell us not to attempt to visualize the epiglottis when epiglottitis is suspected. While I agree with the gist of this warning, I make two minor exceptions: (1) There is no harm when epiglottitis is strongly suspected in a youngster with no or minimal respiratory distress in asking the child to open his or her mouth to allow you to peer at the pharynx with a flashlight. If you see a swollen epiglottitis, the diagnosis is made and you have avoided the quandary that arises on some occasions between immediate intubation and radiographic confirmation. (2) On the other end of the spectrum, you will see some children who fulfill all the clinical criteria for croup, yet you maintain a nagging worry about the remote possibility of epiglottitis. In these situations, you can comfortably use a tongue depressor if necessary and attempt to view a normal epiglottis. Again, one peek may resolve all the issues without costly and time-consuming ancillary studies or therapeutic misadventures.

A 6-year-old girl complains that she has had difficulty urinating for 2 days. Her mother has noted no fever or signs of systemic illness. As an infant, the patient was admitted to the hospital once for pyelonephritis and again for cellulitis that complicated a severe case of chicken pox. Subsequently, her mother reports that she had "normal X-rays" of her kidneys. She is afebrile and appears generally well on examination, except as shown.

1. This problem is the result of:
    A. Exposure to another child
    B. Abuse by an adult
    C. Mechanical irritation
    D. Contact with a fomite
    E. Poor hygiene

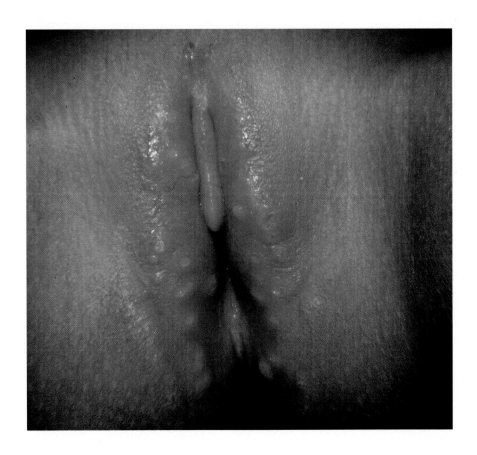

DISCUSSION

ANSWER:

1. **B. Abuse by an adult**

1. The child has genital herpes, probably due to herpes simplex virus (HSV) type 2, and has suffered from sexual abuse. The localized vesicles on an erythematous base are characteristic of this infection. While genital HSV may occasionally result from auto-inoculation in children, this mode of transmission generally occurs in boys between the ages of 1 and 4 years. You must rule out sexual abuse in the prepubertal girl, particularly after 5 years of age. Genital HSV does not spread from child to child or by contact with a fomite (e.g., toilet seat) under ordinary circumstances. Other diseases that you might consider include varicella, which often involves the genitalia but only late in the disease with diffuse truncal lesions, or monilia, which is not vesicular and affects predominantly children in diapers or girls in the immediate prepubertal period. Poor hygiene or mechanical irritation are unlikely explanations and, while they might account for some erythema, would not cause vesicles.

Further Discussion

Upon diagnosing genital HSV in a girl this age, one should involve the appropriate social service agencies. As stated above, the high likelihood of abuse mandates a thorough investigation. While the clinical diagnosis may be obvious, a culture is important from the medicolegal standpoint. HSV 2 is more likely than HSV 1 to be transmitted sexually and, in this day and age, the potential exists for specific DNA matching of viruses from the patient and any alleged perpetrator. In addition to an HSV culture, one should test for *Neisseria gonorrhoeae*, *Chlamydia trachomatis*, and syphilis. Additionally, one might investigate the parents' feeling about serology for HIV. Oral acyclovir will shorten this girl's course but, unfortunately, will not prevent latency and recurrences. Some children with HSV will develop urinary retention, due at least in part to dysuria, and the parents should be instructed in this regard.

A 4-week-old boy returns for a second visit, with continued constipation. He was born after a 40-week gestation with a birth weight of 3.7 kg. At a scheduled check-up at 2 weeks of age, he weighed 3.9 kg; his pediatrician diagnosed reflux and recommended thickened feedings. Six days ago, he was seen because he had not produced a stool for 48 hours. His examination was normal at that time. In the subsequent interval, he had one soft stool. His current weight is 4.0 kg. He is afebrile. Auscultation of his heart reveals a normal sinus rhythm with no murmurs or rubs. His lungs are clear to auscultation. Palpation of the abdomen elicits no tenderness. The liver and spleen are not enlarged, and there are no masses. Bowel sounds are active. His rectal vault contains a minimal amount of soft stool that is guaiac negative. You obtain an X-ray, a complete blood count, and electrolytes.

1. What laboratory findings do you anticipate?
   (See page 47)

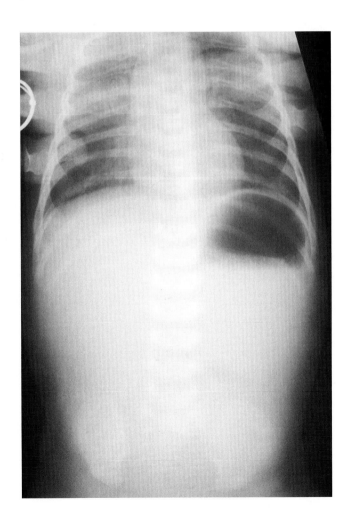

	WBC/mm^3	Bands (%)	Polys (%)	Na (mEq/L)	Cl (mEq/L)	CO$_2$ (mEq/L)
A.	21,000	6	90	131	88	17
B.	14,000	4	78	149	112	19
C.	14,000	2	64	132	84	31
D.	24,000	5	83	135	98	29
E.	12,000	2	59	129	81	14

DISCUSSION

ANSWER:
1. C. 14,000 WBC/mm³; 2% Bands; 64% Polys; 132 mEq/L Na; 84 mEq/L Cl; 31 mEq/L CO_2

1. The X-rays shows a gasless abdomen except for the stomach, indicative of a gastric outlet obstruction. In a 4-week-old, overwhelmingly the most likely diagnosis is pyloric stenosis. Infants with pyloric stenosis vomit large amounts of gastric fluid, which contains high concentrations of hydrogen ions (HCl), sodium, and chloride. While the electrolytes will be normal early in the course, over time a hypochloremic, hyponatremic, alkalosis develops. The WBC count remains normal or may increase slightly, if the infant becomes dehydrated. Only two of the answers indicate alkalosis (bicarbonate of 29 and 31 mEq/L), and only the former of these includes the finding of hypochloremia (84 mEq/L).

Further Discussion

Other causes of obstruction in the first 2 months of life include duodenal atresia, meconium ileus, intussusception, volvulus, and Hirschsprung's disease. Both duodenal atresia and meconium ileus present in the first day or two of life. While duodenal atresia may cause a gasless abdomen, one usually sees a "double-bubble" rather than solitary gastric distension. With intussusception, volvulus, and Hirschsprung's disease, gas would be expected to pass beyond the pylorus into the small bowel. Nonetheless, one would never rule out these emergent conditions solely on the basis of an abdominal radiograph. At this point, an ultrasound would be the study of choice to confirm pyloric stenosis, but an upper gastrointestinal series with barium is a reasonable alternative.

The 14-year-old mother of a 4-month-old female brings her to the emergency department. She says that the baby has had a fever and some diarrhea for 3 days, but offers few additional details despite repeated questioning. Today she reports the child seemed sleepy. The pulse is 160/min, the respiratory rate is 32/min, and the temperature is 38.2°C. The infant's neck is supple. There are no cardiac murmurs and the lungs are clear to auscultation. Palpation of the abdomen elicits no tenderness; stool guaiac is negative. The genitalia are normal.

1. Your initial treatment is:
   A. Ceftriaxone
   B. Hydrocortisone
   C. Gastric intubation
   D. Blood transfusion
   E. Saline

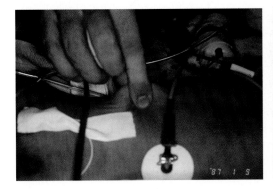 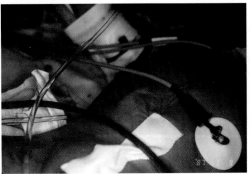

DISCUSSION

ANSWER:

1. E. Saline

1. This infant has tenting of his skin, a sign of severe dehydration. Your initial therapy is normal saline. While the history suggests gastroenteritis, an etiologic diagnosis is less important than prompt rehydration. Since the infant is febrile and ill appearing, administration of a broad spectrum antibiotic, such as ceftriaxone, is reasonable but takes a back seat to the saline. With a scaphoid abdomen and no vomiting, gastrointestinal obstruction seems highly improbable; thus, gastric intubation is not indicated. In the absence of a history of trauma or gastrointestinal bleeding, there is no call for immediate transfusion. Hydrocortisone would be indicated for an infant with congenital adrenal hyperplasia (CAH), which may cause severe dehydration, but usually during the first month of life and often in an infant with ambiguous genitalia.

Further Discussion

The assessment of dehydration in children is an art rather than a science. In general, children who are <5% dehydrated will have only tachycardia and perhaps dry mucous membranes. As dehydration reaches the 10% range, the pulse increases further, skin turgor becomes noticeably decreased, and the mucous membranes are often parched. Above 10% dehydration, one may observe tenting of the skin and hypotension. The laboratory provides little assistance in most cases. Children may be moderately to severely dehydrated with relatively normal electrolytes, and because children who are ill often consume minimal or no protein, the blood urea nitrogen (BUN) frequently does not rise until dehydration becomes severe.

To treat moderate to severe dehydration, establish intravenous access and administer a bolus of 20 cc/kg of saline as rapidly as possible (i.e., within 15 to 30 minutes). Further fluids are titrated against the response in terms of vital signs, mental status, and perfusion. If a child does not improve after an initial bolus, repeat it. For the patient who responds, begin 5% dextrose in either $\frac{1}{2}$ or $\frac{1}{4}$ normal saline at 1.5x to 2x maintenance rate (maintenance: 100 cc/kg for the first 10 kg; 50 cc/kg for the next 10 kg; 20 cc/kg thereafter). As soon as possible, adjust the composition of the fluids based on the results of the patient's electrolyte levels.

During January, a 5-month-old infant comes to the emergency department with respiratory distress. He is well saturated in room air. You hear a few wheezes and crackles, but no heart murmur, feel a liver edge just below the right costal margin, and send him for a chest radiograph. Cardiomegaly is noted and you obtain the following EKG.

1. The most likely diagnosis is congestive heart failure secondary to:
   A. Ventricular septal defect
   B. Aortic stenosis
   C. Cardiomyopathy
   D. Myocarditis
   E. Myocardial infarction

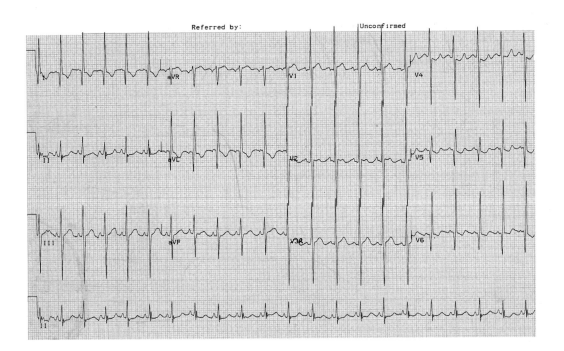

DISCUSSION

ANSWER:
1. E. Myocardial infarction

1. Did your senior resident ever tell you, "All that wheezes is not asthma?" This patient appears to be in mild congestive heart failure without cyanosis, decreasing the probability of many types of cyanotic congenital heart disease. Patients with ventricular septal defects usually have a loud harsh holosystolic murmur and their EKG shows left ventricular hypertrophy. Those with aortic stenosis causing congestive heart failure have systolic ejection murmurs and may also have systolic thrills, a narrowly split or single S2, or a systolic ejection click appreciated over the aortic area (right upper sternal border). The EKG may be normal, show ST-T wave abnormalities, or have signs of left ventricular hypertrophy. In congenital cardiomyopathies, such as endocardial fibroelastosis or storage diseases, murmurs may be absent unless the left ventricular hypertrophy has caused mitral insufficiency. The EKG shows left or biventricular hypertrophy. Acquired myocarditis may present without a murmur and the EKG is quite nonspecific. The EKG may be normal or demonstrate T wave abnormalities, low QRS amplitudes (less than 5 mm in all six limb leads), prolonged PR or QTc intervals, or dysrhythmias. This EKG shows deep Q waves in leads I, AVL, V5 and V6 along with inverted T waves in leads I and AVL, consistent with a lateral myocardial infarct.

Further Discussion

Myocardial infarctions in neonates and young infants can be associated with congenital heart disease, such as aortic stenosis, but in this situation the infarction usually occurs later in life. Neonates with structurally normal hearts and coronary arteries may have infarctions, usually due to thromboembolism that is possibly associated with umbilical vein catheterization, renal vein thrombosis or perinatal asphyxia. This patient had an anomalous origin of the left coronary artery as the cause of his infarction. Of the reported cases of this anomaly, many are thought to have bronchiolitis or other respiratory disease until the chest radiograph suggests another etiology.

The mother of a 3-year-old boy comes home from work to find her son uncomfortable and scratching at his groin. The babysitter reports she observed nothing unusual during the day. Upon taking the boy to the bathroom, the mother noticed swelling of his penis. His past medical history indicates that he was circumcised as a newborn. Currently, he is afebrile. His general examination is normal. Closer inspection of his genitalia is notable for a yellow discharge from his urethra.

1. Your diagnosis is:
   A. Allergic reaction
   B. Hair tourniquet
   C. Paraphimosis
   D. Penile venereal edema
   E. Phimosis

2. Your treatment is:
   A. Manual reduction
   B. Surgical correction
   C. Antibiotic therapy
   D. Diphenhydramine
   E. Aspiration

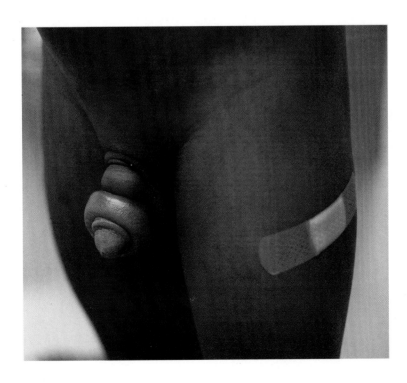

DISCUSSION

ANSWER:
1. D. Penile venereal edema
2. C. Antibiotic therapy

1. Judging solely from the appearance, without the benefit of history or a closer inspection of the phallus, this boy's problem could be an allergic reaction, a hair tourniquet, paraphimosis, or penile venereal edema. Phimosis, a condition in which the foreskin covers the glans and cannot be reduced, is not a possibility. The reciprocal condition, paraphimosis cannot occur in a properly circumcised male. Although a tourniquet may not be obvious from afar, the failure of a careful examination to identify an encircling hair speaks against this entity. Allergic reactions, most frequently secondary to the bite of an insect, may produce a fairly pronounced swelling of the loose tissue of the shaft of the penis, but do not lead to a urethral discharge. Thus we are left with penile venereal edema, which occurs secondary to gonococcal urethritis.

2. Therapy requires an antibiotic effective against *Neisseria gonorrhoeae*. Phimosis in a young boy is generally a physiologic condition needing no treatment. Both paraphimosis and hair tourniquets require prompt correction. Manual reduction suffices to reduce over 95% of paraphimoses, but occasionally a dorsal slit must be made in the prepuce. To correct a hair tourniquet syndrome, the offending strand should be unraveled or cut, taking care to completely remove all loops. Allergic reactions resolve spontaneously and never restrict the flow of urine, but an antihistamine may be prescribed.

Further Discussion

This is an unusual case in several regards. First, sexual abuse, in this case involving fellatio by a female babysitter, more often is perpetrated by males, with young girls as the victims. Second, penile venereal edema is an infrequent complication of gonorrhea. However, as proven by this case, both do occur.

Penile venereal edema is a painless swelling of the shaft of the penis just proximal to the glans in a patient infected with *Neisseria gonorrhoeae*. Standard treatment regimens for gonorrhea lead to prompt resolution. The presence of a Band-Aid on this child's thigh provides a clue to the choice of therapy here: intramuscular ceftriaxone.

A 5-year-old child lacerates his index finger on a jagged piece of metal. He is able to flex and extend the digit at both the proximal and distal interphalangeal joint. Capillary refill over the distal phalanx is brisk. You are unable to gain sufficient cooperation for testing two point discrimination, but the child withdraws to pain.

1. With tourniquet control and wearing magnifying loupes, you carefully explore the wound, specifically attempting to identify an injury to the:
   A. Extensor digitorum
   B. Extensor policis brevis
   C. Flexor digitorum superficialis
   D. Digital artery
   E. Lumbrical muscle

2. You should worry about ischemia to the tissues in this situation if your exploration and repair require more than:
   A. 2 minutes
   B. 5 minutes
   C. 10 minutes
   D. 15 minutes
   E. 20 minutes

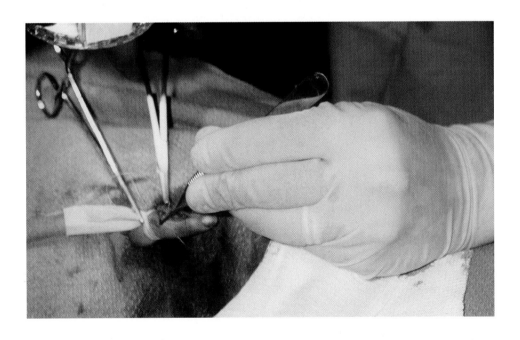

DISCUSSION

ANSWERS:
1. A. **Extensor digitorum**
2. E. **20 minutes**

1. The laceration is located on the dorsal aspect of one of the fingers, in the area where it might involve the extensor digitorum. The extensor policis brevis extends the thumb, and the flexor digitorum superificialis lies on the palmar aspect of the digit. The digital artery is located laterally, and the lumbrical muscle inserts proximal to this wound.

2. If you are worried about ischemia, you need to practice your suturing. Repair of this laceration should require only 15 or 20 minutes, while you could safely leave the tourniquet on for more than half an hour.

Further Discussion

Repair of lacerations of the hand requires a meticulous effort to identify injuries to tendons, vessels, nerves, the nailbed, and the joint capsule. A prerequisite to repair is a knowledge of the anatomy followed by thorough neurovascular evaluation and careful exploration. To facilitate exploration, I strongly recommend that one use loupes and gain hemostasis with a tourniquet. Appropriate follow up is important, as a partial tendon laceration may be missed occasionally, even by an experienced operator.

A 2-year-old child, who recently returned to New York from a visit to Jamaica where he was born, has had a fever and a cough for 3 days. The child's immunizations were complete up to the age of 6 months, but he has not had any subsequent well child care. His temperature is 39°C, pulse 140/min, respirations 44/min, and blood pressure 95/55 mm Hg. He appears somewhat small for his age, apathetic, and in mild respiratory distress. Breath sounds are decreased over the right hemithorax. The heart sounds are normal; a grade 2/6 systolic ejection murmur is appreciated. His abdomen is soft and nontender.

1. The best test to make a specific diagnosis is a:
   A. Culture of sputum
   B. Acid fast stain of gastric washes
   C. Silver stain of bronchoalveolar secretions
   D. Culture of pleural fluid
   E. Echocardiogram

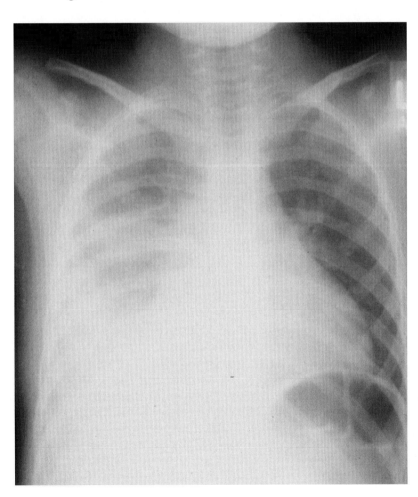

DISCUSSION

ANSWER:

1. **D. Culture of pleural fluid**

1. The X-rays show an infiltrate in the right lung and a pleural effusion. The cardiac silhouette is normal, as are the bones and the soft tissues. Differential diagnosis includes primarily bacterial pneumonia and tuberculosis. *Pneumocystis carinii* causes pneumonia in children infected with human immunodeficiency virus (HIV), but the infiltrate is usually bilateral and streaky, without a large pleural effusion. Congestive heart failure may cause pleural effusion, but one would expect this to be more often bilateral in the presence of cardiomegaly.

   The best diagnostic study is a thoracentesis followed by staining (Gram and acid fast) and culture of the pleural fluid. Culture is more sensitive and will provide a diagnosis in most cases of tuberculosis, as well as identify many bacterial infections. A young child will rarely expectorate sputum, and neither culture nor Gram stain of this material provides accurate information. Gastric washings are helpful in some cases of tuberculosis, but identification of *M. tuberculosis* can be achieved only with culture (requiring 4-6 weeks) or by PCR (not routinely available), and not with acid fast stain alone. If *P. carinii* were suspected, silver stain of secretions obtained by bronchoalveolar lavage might well be diagnostic. The presence of a grade 2/6 murmur in this febrile 2-year-old with respiratory distress probably represents a flow murmur; given the otherwise normal examination and the absence of cardiomegaly, I see no indication for an echocardiogram.

Further Discussion

Several bacterial pathogens are possible etiologic agents for this child's pneumonia, including *Streptococcus pneumoniae*, *Hemophilus influenzae*, and *Staphylococcus aureus*. Overall, pneumococci cause the majority of bacterial pneumonias in children; however, only a small percentage are accompanied by an effusion. On the contrary, *S. aureus* is responsible for only a small portion of pulmonary infections during childhood, but over 50% of staphylococcal pneumonias have a pleural component. *H. influenzae* probably falls in the middle between the other two pathogens in terms of incidence (given that we don't know the vaccination status) and likelihood of effusion. If this child has sickle cell anemia, about which you should certainly be concerned, *Mycoplasma pneumoniae* joins the list.

A 6-year-old boy complains of abdominal pain for 3 days. He vomited three times earlier in the day, but has had no fever or diarrhea. The last emesis was yellowish-green. His mother states that he has had several similar episodes in the past year. On examination, he is afebrile and in no acute distress. His abdomen appears somewhat distended; palpation elicits mild discomfort, but no focal tenderness or peritoneal signs. As you perform a rectal examination, you encounter a "worm."

1. Treatment is:
   A. Reassurance only
   B. Mebendazole
   C. Thiabendazole
   D. Ketoconazole
   E. Neomycin

2. You are concerned about what potential complication in this child?
   A. Intussusception
   B. Intestinal obstruction
   C. Gastrointestinal hemorrhage
   D. Pancreatitis
   E. Hepatic abscess

3. A surgical consultant wants you sedate the child so she can get a better examination. She tells you her favorite drug, but you wisely caution against it. It is:
   A. Midazolam
   B. Morphine
   C. Pentobarbital
   D. Meperidine
   E. Chloral hydrate

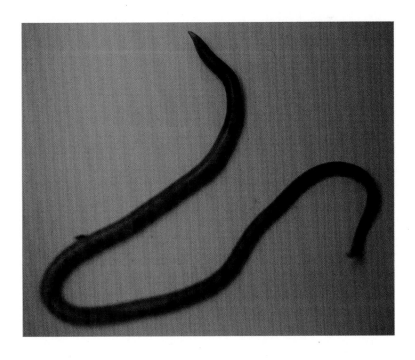

DISCUSSION

ANSWERS:

1. B. Mebendazole
2. B. Intestinal obstruction
3. C. Pentobarbital

1. Mebendazole is the drug of choice for patients who have Ascariasis. Thiabendazole is another anti-helminthic agent, but is not used for this infestation. Ketoconazole sounds similar but works against fungal infections. Neomycin prepares the bowel for surgery, as it is an antibiotic rather than an anti-helminthic agent. Reassurance is all that is needed for whipworm (*Trichuris trichuria*) and would suffice, although not be ideal, for pinworms (*Enterobius vermicularis*), but it is not enough for this child.

2. With a heavy infestation, Ascaris may produce an intestinal obstruction. Hookworms are more likely to cause gastrointestinal bleeding. Hepatic abscesses occur with amebiasis. Pancreatitis is not part of the clinical picture of these helminthic infestations. While polyps and other lesions may serve as a lead point for intussusception, intestinal parasites are not generally implicated.

3. Tell your surgical colleague to avoid pentobarbital, as barbiturates agitate the worms, leading to obstruction. None of the other agents is contraindicated.

Further Discussion

Ascaris lumbricoides commonly infests children in parts of the world other than the United States. This boy had recently arrived in Boston from Honduras, where the problem arose. Ascariasis is seen as well in patients from Puerto Rico. The sighting of Ascaris often provokes fear among the staff in the emergency department. You can reassure your colleagues that the infestation is acquired when the larval form penetrates the sole of the foot.

An 8-year-old boy complains of a rash and swelling of the left side of his neck. His illness began 2 weeks ago with a fever and a lesion on his back, followed shortly thereafter by swelling. Since that time, the fever has resolved but the swelling has increased in size. His past medical history is negative except for "swimmer's ear" on the right 4 weeks ago and "poison ivy" 6 weeks earlier. He denies exposure to kittens.

1. You suspect that the lesion on his back 2 weeks ago was most likely:
   A. A mosquito bite
   B. A thorn scratch
   C. A chancer
   D. A tick bite
   E. Erythema migrans

2. You recommend treatment with:
   A. Streptomycin
   B. Tetracycline
   C. Itraconazole
   D. Penicillin
   E. Chloroquine

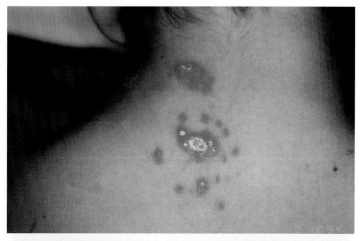

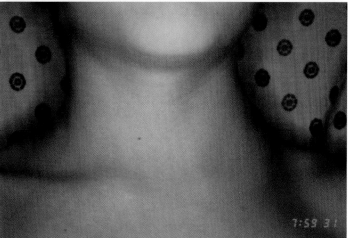

(Photograph courtesy of Marvin Harper, MD)

DISCUSSION

ANSWERS:
1. D. Tick bite
2. A. Streptomycin

1. This boy has tuleremia, which may result from the bite of an animal (raccoon, rabbit, etc.) or a tick. Ticks also transmit Rocky Mountain spotted fever, which causes a generalized maculopapular and then petechial eruption, and Lyme disease, which manifests with erythema migrans (either localized or generalized), which consists of an erythematous macular margin and a central area of clearing. A syphilitic chancer does not resemble this boy's lesion and would be unlikely to occur either in an 8-year-old child or on the back. Mosquitos, particularly in the tropics, transmit malaria but not tularemia. Sporotrichosis, a fungal infection, develops after inoculation from a scratch or puncture wound with a thorn. It almost always involves the distal extremities and causes a linear distribution of nodular lesions without particularly prominent lymph node enlargement.

2. The treatment of choice for tularemia is streptomycin, while gentamicin serves as an alternative. Although appropriate therapies for Rocky Mountain spotted fever, neither tetracycline nor chloramphenicol are very effective for tularemia, as they are only bacteriostatic for this organism. Itraconazole provide excellent therapy for sporotrichosis. Both Lyme disease and syphilis respond to penicillin, used orally for the former, when localized, and intramuscularly for the latter, in uncomplicated cases. Chloroquine is a treatment for malaria, when the parasite is susceptible.

Further Discussion

While tularemia is not a common illness, several thousand cases occur annually in the United States. About half of the patients come from rural areas. Clinical syndromes include ulceroglandular, glandular, oculoglandular, pharyngeal, typhoidal, and pneumonic. This patient suffered from ulceroglandular tularemia, consisting of an ulcerated skin lesion and regional lymphadenopathy. The skin lesion begins as a papule, which enlarges and then ulcerates; multiple lesions may occur. The ulcers take weeks to heal. With animal bites, the initial lesion usually affects the extremities, while truncal involvement is seen more frequently following transmission by ticks. Cervical adenopathy is most common in children.

A 15-year-old boy, seen in August, complains of a rash for 2 months over the summer. He denies recent illnesses and states that the rash in not pruritic. On examination, he is afebrile and appears in good general health.

1. You find the following positive laboratory test:
    A. VDRL titer
    B. KOH preparation
    C. Anti-nuclear antibody
    D. Viral culture
    E. None of the above

2. Your therapy is:
    A. Benzathine penicillin
    B. Mycostatin
    C. Acyclovir
    D. Diphenhydramine
    E. Selenium sulfide

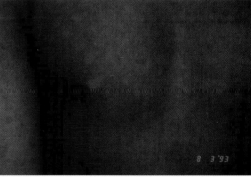

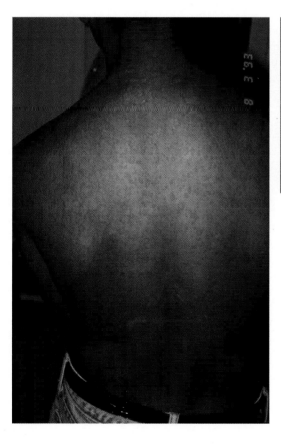

DISCUSSION

ANSWERS:
1. **B. KOH preparation**
2. **E. Selenium sulfide**

1. Usually, tinea versicolor is diagnosed on the basis of clinical appearance. When confirmation is needed, microscopic examination of a KOH preparation from a skin scraping reveals the causative organism, *Pityrosporum obiculare*, in clusters of large spores and short, stubby hyphae, referred to as "meatballs and spaghetti." Rashes with a similar appearance include pityriasis rosea and secondary syphilis. Pityriasis rosea is presumed to be of viral etiology, but no specific agent has been identified and neither culture nor serology is helpful. A positive VDRL is found in secondary syphilis. Lupus is unusual in a male and, while the rash may be photosensitive and accentuated by sun exposure in the summer, it does not usually affect the trunk so much as the face.

2. The treatment for tinea versicolor is topical selenium sulfide. After wetting the skin, shampoo is applied over the entire body and the lather is left on for 20 minutes. Although mycostatin is an antifungal agent, it is not used for this disease. Benzathine penicillin, given as once weekly injections, treats secondary syphilis. While no therapy cures pityriasis rosea, diphenhydramine or other antipruritic agents may be prescribed for symptomatic relief. The antiviral drug, acyclovir, has no role in any of these conditions.

Further Discussion

The diagnosis of tinea versicolor is often overlooked. Clues include chronicity (months to years), exacerbation after exposure to sunlight, and the characteristic hypo- and hyperpigmented macules. By way of contrast, both pityriasis rosea and secondary syphilis resolve spontaneously after 4-6 weeks and manifest as a papulosquamous eruption.

An 11-year-old falls 10 feet from a rope in gym class and complains of pain in the right forearm. Other than tenderness in the area of complaint, his examination is normal.

1. The most appropriate treatment is:
   A. Elastic bandage
   B. Splint
   C. Cast
   D. Closed reduction
   E. Open reduction

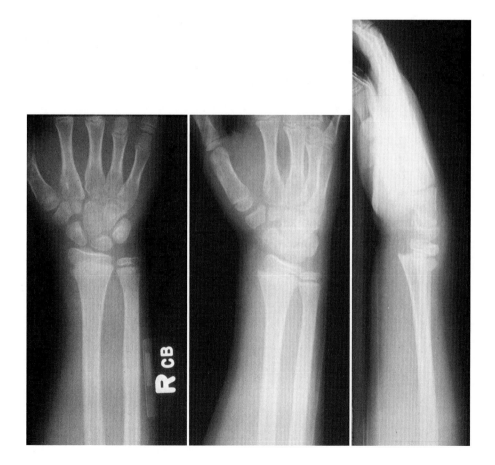

DISCUSSION

ANSWER:

1. **D. Closed reduction**

1. This boy, the son of one of the editors, sustained a displaced Salter II fracture of the distal radius. It is difficult to visualize the small metaphyseal fragment, which distinguishes a Salter I from a Salter II. The treatment, however is the same. Reduction of the fracture is mandatory and accomplished readily by manipulation in the emergency department under adequate sedation. In this case, nitrous oxide was administered, but ketamine or fentanyl/midazolam represent reasonable alternatives. An elastic bandage would not provide sufficient immobilization and might well cause problems as the swelling increased over the first 48 hours. Casting without reduction is contraindicated, and an open reduction is not necessary. A displaced physeal injury should not be simply splinted and referred without orthopedic consultation.

Further Discussion

As compared to adults, children sustain a number of unique injuries including: (1) physeal fractures, (2) torus or buckle fractures, (3) greenstick fractures, (4) bowing deformities, and (5) avulsion fractures. Approximately 20% of pediatric fractures involve the physis (growth plate), occurring through the zone of provisional calcification, a relatively weak area of the germinal growth plate. The majority of these injuries involve the radius or ulna. The most frequently used classification system is that proposed by Salter and Harris. Probably the most important point to keep in mind is that positive physical findings, such as point tenderness and swelling over the physis, in the face of a negative radiograph suggest a Salter Harris I fracture which requires proper immobilization.

An 8-year-old previously healthy girl complains of a sore throat and low-grade fever for 2 days. She has also had a headache. On examination, her temperature is 38.3°C and her pulse is 110/min. Abnormal findings are shown in the pictures.

1. Appropriate treatment for this condition is:
   A. Acyclovir
   B. Penicillin
   C. Ribavirin
   D. Reassurance
   E. Amoxicillin

2. A potential complication with this organism is:
   A. Rheumatic fever
   B. Keratoconjunctivitis
   C. Pelvic inflammatory disease
   D. Peritonsillar abscess
   E. Myocarditis

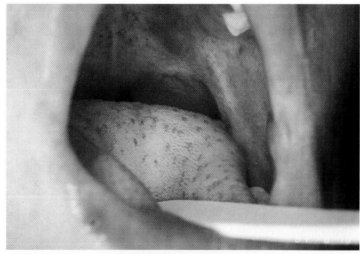

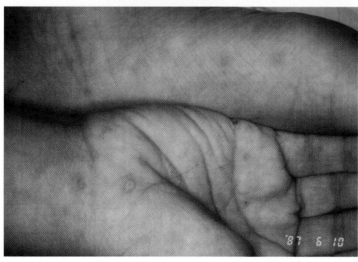

DISCUSSION

ANSWERS:

1. **D. Reassurance**
2. **E. Myocarditis**

1. This girl has Hand-Foot-Mouth disease due to Coxsackie virus, which resolves in 3-5 days without treatment. Other causes of infections in the oral cavity are Herpes simplex virus (HSV), Group A *Streptococcus*, and *Neisseria gonorrhoeae.* Stomatitis due to HSV usually involves the anterior buccal mucosa and lips, rather than the palate. While stomatitis occasionally causes localized lesions on a finger or thumb (herpetic whitlow), the vesicles are grouped, as opposed to isolated, and do not appear on both hands or on the hands and the feet. In selected circumstances, acyclovir has a role with HSV. Ribavirin is recommended by some authorities for RSV infections in compromised hosts or of usual severity. Both amoxicillin and penicillin treat streptococcal pharyngitis. Group A *Streptococcus* may very rarely produce a blistering distal dactylitis of the hands; as with HSV, the lesions do not diffusely involve the hands and feet.

2. Coxsackie viruses cause Hand-Foot-Mouth disease, herpangina, and myocarditis. While one of the type A Coxsackie viruses (A16) causes Hand-Foot-Mouth disease, and the type B agents are more commonly isolated from patients with myocarditis, type A agents may involve the heart as well. Group A streptococcal infection may lead to either nonsuppurative complications (acute rheumatic fever, glomerulonephritis) or suppurative sequelae (peritonsillar abscess). HSV causes keratoconjunctivitis, and the gonococcus (an occasional pharyngeal pathogen) is implicated in about one-third of the cases of pelvic inflammatory disease.

Further Discussion

Patients with Hand-Foot-Mouth disease have findings that are sufficiently characteristic for a clinical diagnosis. Neither viral nor bacterial (to exclude streptococcal disease) cultures are indicated. The majority of patients require no therapy beyond an antipyretic. Unlike herpetic stomatitis, the lesions rarely interfere with hydration. Perhaps a minor point, I usually avoid telling parents the specific name of this infection, as they usually confuse it with a veterinary disease and become quite anxious.

This young man injured his knee while jumping on a trampoline.

1. Your diagnosis is:
   A. Acute hemarthrosis
   B. Distal femur fracture
   C. Dislocated patella
   D. Patellar fracture
   E. Torn medial meniscus

2. To treat this problem, you should:
   A. Consult an orthopedist
   B. Extend the leg
   C. Place a knee immobilizer
   D. Aspirate the joint
   E. Apply a long leg cast

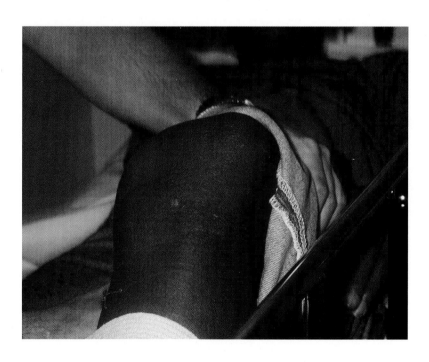

DISCUSSION

ANSWERS:
1. C. Dislocated patella
2. B. Extend the leg

1. The patient seems to be in severe pain, and his patella is displaced laterally. He does not appear to have any other knee deformity. The most likely diagnosis is an acutely dislocated patella, which is frequently seen in patients without any direct trauma to the patella. Acute hemarthroses accompany fractures of the knee, which extend into the joint, and meniscal or ligamentous injuries. These injuries would cause generalized knee swelling. Distal femur fractures are caused by severe direct trauma and may lead to knee deformity and extensive swelling proximal to the knee. A patellar fracture is usually caused by direct trauma and produces generalized knee swelling and a high riding patella, rather than one displaced laterally.

2. A patellar dislocation should be treated by immediate reduction. This can be performed in less than 15 seconds and should result in pain reduction. Tell the patient and parents what you are going to do and then quickly extend the leg as you push the patella medially. You will feel and see the patella suddenly move back into place. Post-reduction radiographs (anteroposterior, lateral, and "skyline" or "sunrise" view if possible) should be obtained to determine if an osteochondral fracture of the medial aspect of the patella or lateral femoral condyle fracture is present. A knee immobilizer for 2-4 weeks, followed by physical therapy, is recommended after reduction. Complications include recurrent patellar dislocations and osteochondral fragments that may not be seen on acute radiographs.

Further Discussion

Patellar dislocations are common in older children and adolescents 11 to 18 years of age, and more commonly affect females than males. The majority are lateral dislocations and only 10% follow direct trauma. Most commonly, dislocations are associated with a twisting movement or a fall during activities ranging from gymnastics and cheerleading to dancing or swinging a golf club. When a patellar dislocation is the obvious diagnosis and the patient is suffering significant pain, reduction may precede radiographic evaluation.

This 4-year-old girl is brought to the emergency department by her mother who saw blood in her underwear earlier in the morning. The child and her mother deny trauma, possible placement of a foreign body in her vagina, fever, urinary frequency, dysuria, or diarrhea. No one in the family has renal disease or congenital hearing loss.

1. Which diagnostic study would you order?
    A. Urinalysis
    B. Urine culture
    C. Vaginal cultures
    D. Cystoscopy
    E. None of the above

2. Which treatment would be most likely to help this patient?
    A. Amoxicillin
    B. Estrogen cream
    C. Mebendazole
    D. Surgical excision
    E. Ceftriaxone

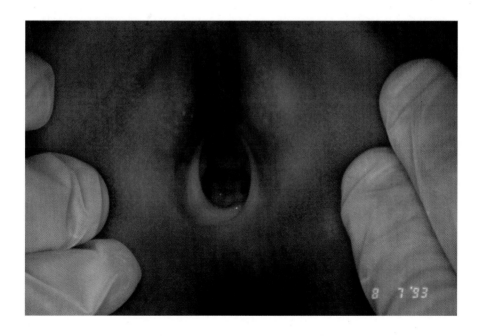

DISCUSSION

ANSWERS:
1. E. None of the above
2. B. Estrogen cream

1. This child requires no diagnostic studies, once you have carefully examined her external genitalia. She has a round, red, annular lesion with a central dimple above her vaginal introitus. This doughnut-shaped mass consists of prolapsed urethral mucosa. The mucosa is red and swollen due to impairment of venous blood flow, and, if not treated, the mucosa may necrose. Occasionally the mass is so large that it occludes the vaginal orifice and the central dimple may be difficult to see. In this case, inserting a catheter into the bladder through the prolapsed urethra would confirm the diagnosis. A urinalysis may have a few red blood cells. A urine culture should be sterile and a vaginal culture should not grow any pathogens. Cystoscopy is not necessary.

2. Although no controlled studies have been performed, a 2-week course of a topical estrogen cream such as Premarin along with sitz baths should improve the problem in most cases. Some experts recommend antiseptic soaps and/or topical or systemic antimicrobials. Complete resolution may be expected in 4-8 weeks. Prolapsed urethras do not usually recur. A gynecology consult should be obtained if the mucosa appears necrotic, as surgical excision within the next few days may be required.

Further Discussion

Blood in a child's underwear could be from a urinary, vaginal or rectal source, and a careful examination of the genitals in the knee-to-chest or supine position is mandatory. If rectal or vulvar excoriations are noted, a scotch tape test for pinworms would be helpful. Vaginal bleeding from a foreign body may present as bleeding with or without a foul-smelling discharge. Young girls frequently place small foreign bodies, such as toilet tissue, in their vaginas. Malignant tumors (sarcoma botryoides) are rare and resemble masses of grape-like lesions. Vaginal polyps are also very rare and appear as smooth pedunculated masses in the vagina. Condyloma acuminatum, caused by the human papilloma virus, may occur in the vagina as well as the rectum, but the mass appears verrucous or fleshy. Neither tumors, polyps nor condyloma should appear as annular or doughnut-shaped masses above the vaginal introitus.

Urethral prolapse occurs in girls between 2 and 10 years of age and in postmenopausal women. The majority of the young patients are African American, and occasionally the children have a history of coughing or constipation that may have increased their intra-abdominal pressure. The exact etiology of this disorder is unknown.

A 16-year-old male presents to the emergency department feeling weak and lethargic. He has vomited for the last 2 days and tells you he used to go the renal clinic at another hospital. Although he looks ill, the rest of his examination is unremarkable. The phlebotomist has sent off a battery of blood tests and the nurse hands you the following EKG.

1. The patient's most likely diagnosis is:
   A. Myocarditis
   B. Ventricular tachycardia
   C. Hyperkalemia
   D. Prolonged QT syndrome
   E. First degree AV block

2. As your evaluation continues, the boy suddenly turns gray. You cannot palpate his pulse. Which of the following is the most specific intervention to provide immediate improvement?
   A. Calcium
   B. Atropine
   C. Lidocaine
   D. Kayexalate
   E. Propranolol

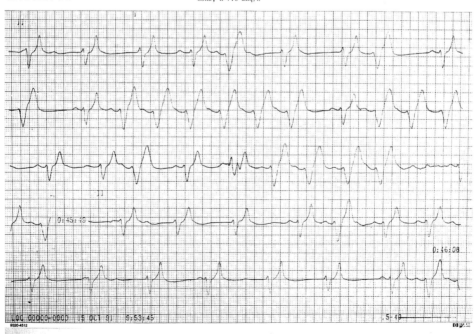

DISCUSSION

ANSWERS:
1. C. Hyperkalemia
2. A. Calcium

1. Although myocarditis may make patients feel weak and lethargic, they are usually tachycardic and have other signs of congestive heart failure such as rales, an S3 gallop and hepatomegaly. Almost any dysrhythmia can be the first sign of myocarditis, but peaked T waves are not characteristic. This patient does have a prolonged QRS complex as seen in ventricular tachycardia, but his heart rate only varies from 45 to 75, too slow for this disorder. While in some leads of the EKG his QT may be a little long, in prolonged QT syndromes the QTc is usually very prolonged (e.g., .55 to .65 seconds). The PR interval is about .2 seconds, just at the upper limit of normal, and might be due to first degree heart block or secondary to another condition that explains the other EKG abnormalities seen here as well.

   The most remarkable abnormality on this EKG is the presence of very tall, peaked T waves. This finding may occur with left ventricular hypertrophy, myocardial infarctions, cerebrovascular accidents and hyperkalemia. Although examination of lead II cannot rule out the first two conditions, it does not support either diagnosis. The patient's lack of headache or focal motor deficits rules out a cerebrovascular accident. Tall T waves, a long PR interval, and a wide QRS duration are all consistent with hyperkalemia, as is his history of attendance at a renal clinic.

2. For symptomatic patients with cardiac arrhythmias or a potassium level greater than 8.0 mEq/L, intravenous calcium, under continuous EKG monitoring may be used. Calcium reduces the membrane excitability induced by hyperkalemia within minutes. This effect is transient so that other therapies, such as glucose, sodium bicarbonate, and kayexalate need to be initiated. The combination of glucose and insulin, or glucose alone in nondiabetics, drives potassium into cells by increasing endogenous insulin. This lowers plasma potassium. Sodium bicarbonate raises the pH and also drives potassium into cells. Both therapies decrease potassium levels within 30 minutes. Kayexalate, a cation exchange resin, absorbs potassium and releases sodium in the gut, therefore removing potassium from the body over a few hours. Peritoneal dialysis also removes potassium, but it may take hours to arrange the procedure. Lidocaine may be used for ventricular tachycardia, and atropine in heart block. Therapy for patients with prolonged QT syndromes may include beta blockers.

CASE 32

The mother of this 10-day-old boy brings him to be evaluated for a discharge from his left nipple that she noticed for the first time several hours ago. The child was born by normal spontaneous vaginal delivery after a term, uncomplicated gestation. He left the hospital on day 2 and has been doing well. The temperature is 37.6°C rectally. Examination of the HEENT (head, eyes, ears, nose, and throat) is normal. Breath sounds are clear in all lobes. The heart rate is 140/min, and no murmurs are heard. The liver is palpable 1 cm below the right costal margin and the spleen is 2 cm below the left costal margin.

1. Appropriate management includes:
   A. Reassurance
   B. Oral cephalexin
   C. Intravenous ampicillin and
      gentamicin
   D. Incision and drainage
   E. Warm compresses

2. The cause of the problem is:
   A. Bacterial
   B. Allergic
   C. Hormonal
   D. Traumatic
   E. Nutritional

3. This condition, properly treated, may have the following outcome in some children:
   A. Persistence
   B. Recurrence in childhood
   C. Systemic spread
   D. Sequelae at puberty
   E. None of the above

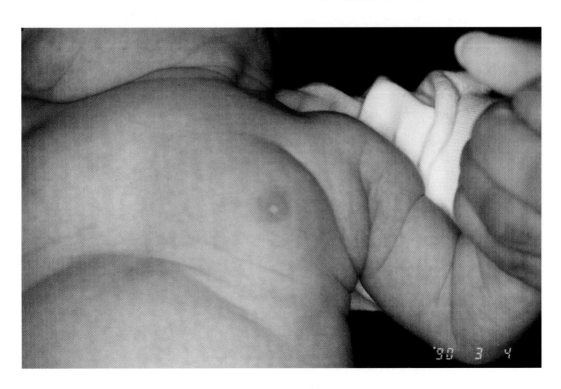

DISCUSSION

ANSWERS:
1. A. Reassurance
2. C. Hormonal
3. E. None of the above

1. This baby has a pubertal gynecomastia which occurs normally in infants. In addition to enlarging, the breast bud may produce secretions, known as "witch's milk." No treatment is indicated; even benign measures, such as warm compresses, play no role. The swelling subsides, depending on the degree of stimulation, in 2-6 weeks. Manipulation, performed ill-advisedly by some parents in an effort to "milk" the secretions out of the breast bud, may lead to infection. Surgical therapy is contraindicated, as it is totally unnecessary and carries risks, particularly for females.

2. Maternal hormones cross the placenta and may stimulate the breast tissue in both males and females. While infection may produce a mastitis, this breast is not erythematous and the discharge is not purulent. Trauma and allergic reactions may produce swelling, but are highly unlikely to affect the breast of a neonate. Nutritional factors have no role.

3. Watchful waiting results in complete resolution with no complications whatsoever. The gynecomastia does not recur once the hormones have been cleared and the swelling resolves. Incision and drainage, if done because self-limited enlargement of the breast tissue is confused with an abscess, has the potential to injure the breast bud and produce a serious cosmetic problem for girls at the time of puberty.

Further Discussion

Breast lesions are common at two times during childhood: the neonatal period and early puberty. Both neonatal gynecomastia and mastitis affect newborns. In girls, the development of a breast bud as early as 8-years-old marks the onset of puberty; prior to this age breast bud development suggests premature thelarche or, if accompanied by the appearance of other secondary sexual characteristics, precocious puberty. Boys may seek reassurance that a pubertal gynecomastia is normal and self-limited.

A previously healthy 2-year-old girl is brought to the emergency department at your community hospital by her father who found her with a half empty bottle of medicine, which had been prescribed to help curb "bed-wetting" in a 5-year-old brother. You estimate the child's weight at 10-12 kg. She appears lethargic and has a respiratory rate of 34/min. Her pulse is rapid and thready to palpation. The oxygen saturation is 96%.

1. Your initial management includes:
    A. Defibrillation
    B. Naloxone
    C. Adenosine
    D. Bicarbonate
    E. Procainamide

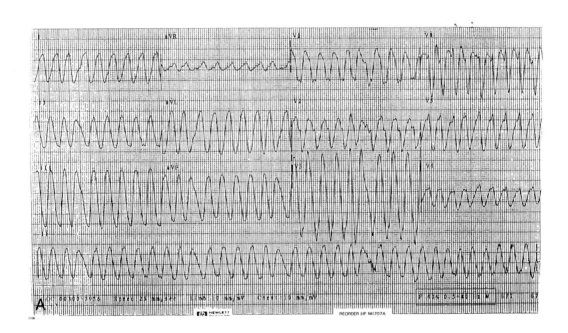

You treat the patient with 10 mEq of sodium bicarbonate intravenously. Her response is shown below.

2. This girl most likely ingested:
   A. Phenytoin
   B. Digoxin
   C. Imipramine
   D. Diltiazam
   E. Theophylline

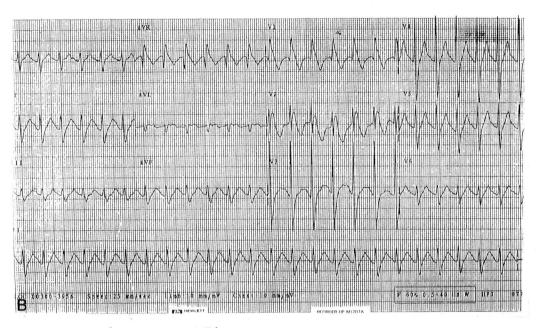

(EKG courtesy of Susan Torrey, MD)

DISCUSSION

ANSWERS:

2. C. Imipramine
1. D. Bicarbonate

(Editor's Note: Answers are reversed to facilitate the discussion.)

2. This patient ingested imipramine, a tricyclic antidepressant that causes widening of the QRS complex in overdoses and, in higher doses, ventricular tachycardia or fibrillation. The intended use of the medication, the curtailment of enuresis, provides a clue to the identity in addition to the findings on the EKG, as imipramine is the only drug on the list prescribed for this indication. Toxicity from digoxin, used for congestive heart failure, manifests predominantly as heart block and atrioventricular dissociation. Overdosage of another drug used to treat cardiovascular disorders, diltiazem, leads to hypotension, bradycardia, and heart block. Ingestion of phenytoin produces primarily neurologic signs and hypotension. At very high blood levels, usually in excess of 100 μg/ml, theophylline may lead to rhythm disturbances, including supraventricular and ventricular tachycardia.

1. In patients with cardiac toxicity from the ingestion of a tricyclic antidepressant, alkalinization specifically antagonizes these effects. If the patient was in extremis and did not respond to alkalinization, you could start with cardioversion, rather than defibrillation. Adenosine is the drug of choice for supraventricular tachycardia but will not work for ventricular tachycardia. While procainamide is an effective treatment for ventricular tachycardia resistant to other therapies, it is not a first choice and must be administered slowly, which limits its utility for an acutely ill patient. Naloxone antagonizes narcotics, which cause respiratory depression primarily and arrhythmias only with hypoxia; here the saturation was 96%.

Further Discussion

Ingestion of a tricyclic antidepressant by a child should be considered a potentially serious event. As little as 10-20 mg/kg of most tricyclic agents represents a moderate to serious exposure, with the potential for coma and cardiovascular symptoms. Fatalities are likely when 35-50 mg/kg is ingested. These drugs have anticholinergic activity as well as "quinidine-like" effects that depress myocardial conduction and may lead to premature ventricular contractions and ventricular tachycardia, particularly torsades de pointes.

This teenager was struck by a car. He was intubated at the scene and had a large-bore intravenous catheter placed by paramedics. On arrival to the emergency department he is unresponsive and intubated, and his cervical spine is immobilized. His pulse is 160/min, respiratory rate bagged is 24/min, blood pressure is 95/60 mm Hg, and his oxygen saturation, on 100% oxygen, is 100%. The trachea is midline, breath sounds are decreased on the left, heart sounds are present, the abdomen seems soft, and the left thigh is swollen and deformed. His pupils are equal, round, and reactive to light, and his Glasgow Coma Scale is 6 (eyes do not open to painful stimuli, he withdraws to painful stimuli and does not cough despite the endotracheal tube). A second large-bore intravenous catheter is placed and a spun hematocrit is 29%. The stat portable chest X-ray is shown.

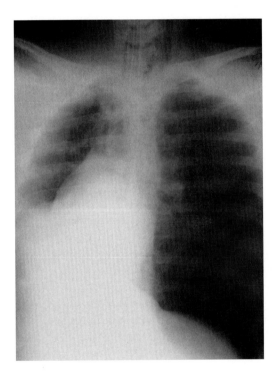

1. Your next procedure is:
   A. Thoracostomy tube placement
   B. Transfusion of packed red blood cells
   C. Pericardiocentesis
   D. Repositioning the endotracheal tube
   E. A page to the on-call surgeon

2. While the necessary equipment is being obtained, the nurse tells you that she can no longer palpate a pulse, although the EKG monitor still shows a sinus tachycardia. You should immediately begin CPR and:
   A. Bolus with 1 mg/kg of lidocaine
   B. Perform a pericardiocentesis
   C. Perform a needle thoracentesis
   D. Give epinephrine 1 mg intravenously
   E. Move the patient to the operating room

DISCUSSION

ANSWERS:
1. A. Thoracostomy tube placement
2. C. Perform a needle thoracentesis

1. The chest radiograph shows a large left tension pneumothorax with the heart deviated to the right. The endotracheal tube is in good position and a nasogastric tube is in place. The affected lung is collapsed, the contralateral lung is compressed and the vena cava is displaced. The collapsed lung is caused by a one-way air leak from the lungs to the pleural space. The combination of impaired ventilation and decreased venous return leads to decreased cardiac output and constitutes a life-threatening emergency. Your response should be immediate placement of a thoracostomy tube. A needle thoracentesis would provide temporary relief if the patient were to deteriorate either clinically or in terms of oxygen saturation. The patient's hematocrit is low, but transfusion of packed red blood cells will not reverse the impaired ventilation and hypotension. Although the signs of cardiac tamponade and tension pneumothorax may be similar (tachycardia, hypotension, cyanosis, and distended neck veins) the radiograph confirms the tension pneumothorax and pericardiocentesis should not be attempted now. Decreased breath sounds on the left may be due to a right mainstem bronchus intubation, but this radiograph does not show right lung hyperinflation. This patient needs to be stabilized before being transferred to the operating room.

2. The lack of a pulse with electrical activity on EKG is called pulseless electrical activity (PEA) or electromechanical dissociation. Cardiac ultrasound studies in adults with PEA have demonstrated that almost 90% have synchronous myocardial wall motion, suggesting that the lack of a palpable pulse is due to inadequate, not absent, myocardial contraction. Tension pneumothorax is a well known cause of PEA. Neither lidocaine nor epinephrine will restore a peripheral pulse, as the patient needs immediate needle thoracentesis followed by thoracostomy tube placement. Cardiac tamponade can also cause PEA, but the radiograph clearly shows a tension pneumothorax. If the patient remained in PEA after chest tube placement and intravascular volume resuscitation then cardiac tamponade should be reconsidered, along with treatment of acidosis, hypothermia, hyperkalemia, and certain drug overdoses (tricyclic antidepressants, digitalis, beta blockers and calcium channel blockers).

Further Discussion

Once the chest tube tray is opened and fluid resuscitation has begun, rapidly prepare the skin at the anterior axillary line in the fifth intercostal space, which can be quickly identified at the nipple level anterior to the midaxillary line. If the patient is awake, anesthetize the skin and rib periosteum. Make a 3 cm horizonal incision and bluntly dissect through the subcutaneous tissue just over the rib (to avoid the neurovascular bundle inferior to the rib). Puncture the parietal pleura with a clamp. You may hear or feel air rushing out. Place your finger into the tract to verify your position. Holding the thoracostomy tube with a clamp just proximal to the tip of the tube, advance it into the pleural space. If correctly placed, you will see "fogging" of the tube and/or hear air flow. Suture the tube in place, apply a dressing, and immediately obtain a chest radiograph. You have just saved a patient's life!

A 9-year-old boy comes to the emergency department in Boston during December for a rash on his foot. He has no systemic symptoms, including fever and malaise. The rash is neither painful nor pruritic. It developed 1 week ago, several days after he returned from a vacation to a Caribbean island.

1. For treatment, you recommend:
    A. Hydrocortisone topically
    B. Permethrin (Elimite®) topically
    C. Thiabendazole orally
    D. Erythromycin orally
    E. Lindane (Kwell®) topically

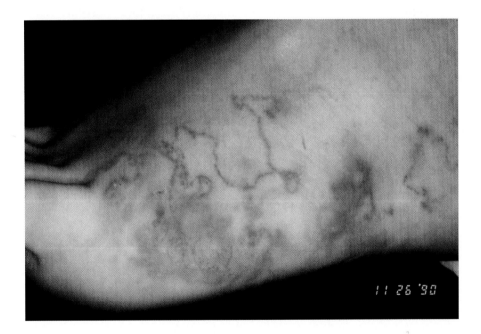

DISCUSSION

ANSWER:

1. C. Thiabendazole orally

1. If you think this rash looks "creepy," then you are on the right track. Known as "creeping eruption" or "creeping hook" in some locales, the condition is cutaneous larval migrans. Treatment consists of thiabendazole, either orally (25 mg/kg twice daily for 2 days) or topically (10% aqueous solution four times daily). Both lindane (Kwell) and permethrin (Elimite) are effective against scabies, but lindane has a lower rate of cure and may be absorbed in quantities sufficient enough to cause seizures. For impetigo, characterized by crusted, bullous, or purulent lesions, oral erythromycin is a drug of choice. Hydrocortisone would be indicated for atopic dermatitis or allergic contact dermatitis, both of which cause an oozing, eczematous eruption.

Further Discussion

Cutaneous larval migrans results from an infestation with *Ancyclostoma braziliense*, the dog and cat hookworm. It is characterized by serpiginous, erythematous, elevated skin lesions. The disease in the United States occurs mostly in the southeast, more often in children than in adults. Diagnosis relies on visual recognition, since biopsy does not usually identify an organism. Perhaps the disease most likely to enter into the differential diagnosis is scabies. Although the lesions of scabies are described as serpiginous in some texts, infestation with this mite more often manifests as papules, excoriations, and in some cases vesicles. Secondary impetiginization is common. Unlike *Ancyclostoma braziliense*, *Sarcoptes scabiei* may be identified in scrapings of the skin.

CASE 36

Parents bring in their 12-year-old Pop Warner football star. He has been complaining of thigh pain and limping for 1 month. A radiograph is obtained.

1. The most likely diagnosis is:
    A. Legg-Calve-Perthes disease
    B. Hip fractures
    C. Transient synovitis
    D. Slipped capital femoral epiphyses
    E. Juvenile rheumatoid arthritis

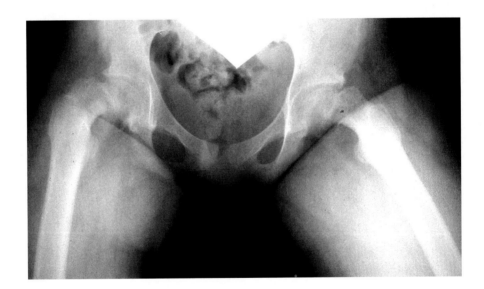

DISCUSSION

ANSWER:

1. C. Slipped capital femoral epiphyses

1. The radiograph shows the femoral heads displaced inferior to the femoral neck, diagnostic of slipped capital femoral epiphyses. An imaginary line running along the superior femoral neck should intersect at least a small part of the femoral head. Hip fractures are rare in children and are seen acutely after severe trauma. Transient synovitis will cause limp, but should have resolved by now and the radiograph should be normal or indicative of a small joint effusion. In Legg-Perthes disease or avascular necrosis of the femoral head, radiographs may be normal or show a widened distance between the ossified femoral head and the acetabulum on the effected side, a less radio-opaque femoral head, or later a flattened femoral head. The early films in juvenile rheumatoid arthritis may be normal or suggest a joint effusion.

Further Discussion

Patients with a slipped capital femoral epiphysis are usually 9- to 16-years-old and are frequently obese, while those with avascular necrosis are usually 4- to 8-years-old and below average height and weight. This patient is unusual since only 10% of affected patients have bilateral involvement. On examination, an affected patient will have pain and limitation of motion of the hip. The involved hip will externally rotate when flexed.

The correct diagnosis may be delayed, which perhaps contributes to a poor outcome, when patients present with unusual symptoms or inadequate radiographs are obtained. 20-30% of patients with slipped capital femoral epiphysis complain of knee or thigh pain since branches of the femoral and obturator nerves innervate the hip, thigh, and knee. Since the anteroposterior view of the hip may be normal, a frog leg lateral should also be obtained.

Therapy is surgical and an orthopedic surgeon should be consulted in a timely fashion.

A 2-year-old boy has lesions on his thumb, which first appeared 5 days ago. His father applied a topical antibiotic cream for 3 days without improvement. Two days ago, the boy's physician prescribed oral amoxicillin-clavulanic acid. Despite continued therapy, the father feels the problem is much worse.

The boy is afebrile. Examination of his HEENT shows no abnormalities. His neck is supple without adenopathy. The lungs are clear, and no cardiac murmurs are auscultated. His abdomen is nontender; the liver and spleen are not palpable. He moves his arms and legs freely. A 1 × 1 cm nontender axillary lymph node is palpable on the side of the lesions on his thumb.

1. Which of the following treatments is contraindicated?
   A. Cephalexin orally
   B. Warm compresses
   C. Mupirocin topically
   D. Acyclovir orally
   E. Incision and drainage

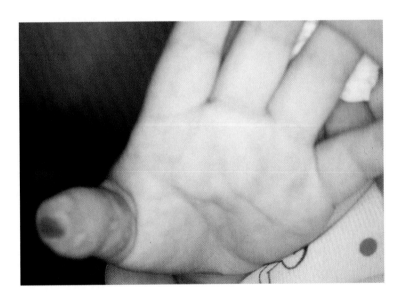

DISCUSSION

ANSWER:

1. **E. Incision and drainage**

1. This boy has a herpetic whitlow. Acyclovir, which is active against herpes simplex, represents a reasonable therapeutic option, although definitive studies on whitlow in children have not been performed. Both topical mupirocin and oral cephalexin are antibacterial agents used for the treatment of impetigo. Warm compress have no effect on the course of whitlow. Finally, incision and drainage is contraindicated, as it offers no therapeutic benefits and may delay resolution.

Further Discussion

Whitlow is much more common than you probably think. I see a case a month. When confronting this diagnosis, I am always reminded of the importance of universal precautions. In the "old days" before widespread use of gloves, whitlow occurred with regularity among physicians, particularly anesthesiologists, who used their exposed digits to pry open the mouths of patients before endotracheal intubation.

A previously healthy 11-year-old boy developed this rash approximately 2 weeks ago. It has been spreading. He has not been febrile or felt ill recently, but his mother is concerned that the problem has not gone away. His temperature is 37.6°C. He has no photophobia, rhinitis, otitis, or pharyngitis. His neck is supple. No murmurs are heard and his lungs are clear to auscultation. He does not have any regional adenopathy. His neurological examination is normal, except the right side of his mouth appears to droop.

1. Appropriate treatment is:
   A. Diphenhydramine orally
   B. Ceftriaxone intravenously
   C. Methylprednisolone intravenously
   D. Amoxicillin orally
   E. Penicillin intravenously

2. You send a number of studies on the blood to the lab and may perform what additional test?
   A. CT of the head
   B. Lumbar puncture
   C. MR of the head
   D. Sinus X-rays
   E. Bone scan

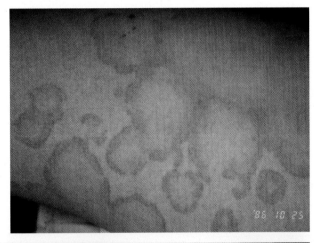

3. His risk of developing arthritis within the next year is:
   A. <2%
   B. 10%
   C. 25%
   D. 40%
   E. >50%

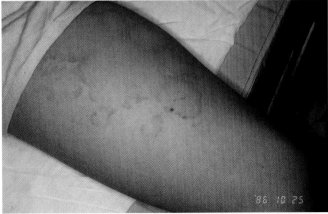

DISCUSSION

ANSWERS:
1. D. Amoxicillin orally
2. B. Lumbar puncture
3. A. <2%

1. The rash is erythema migrans (formerly called erythema chronicum migrans or ECM), which occurs with Lyme disease. Patients who have only cutaneous signs or a combination of erythema chronicum and facial palsy respond to oral therapy with a number of antibiotics, including amoxicillin. Complicated cases, with involvement of the central nervous system or joints, are more appropriately treated with intravenous antibiotics, such as ceftriaxone or penicillin. Either steroids or antihistamines have a potential role in allergic conditions such as urticaria.

2. Although not pictured, this child has a palsy of his right seventh cranial nerve, described here as a facial droop., This finding raises the specter of involvement of the central nervous system (CNS). To diagnose CNS involvement, a lumbar puncture is indicated. Neither CT scans nor MRI play a role, as mass lesions do not occur with Lyme disease. In a case of Bell's palsy with an obvious purulent otitis media, one might consider sinus X-rays to detect mastoiditis; however, there is no such clinical indication in this child. Similarly, neither the rash nor the findings in the region of the ear point to an osteomyelitis which might be detected by bone scan.

3. Chronic arthritis is rare after infection with *Borrelia burgdorferi*, occurring in less than 2% of children.

Further Discussion

The diagnosis of Lyme disease is difficult, as the serologic assays are unreliable. Depending on the laboratory and the methodology, children with definite infections may have negative tests. On the other hand, false-positive results occur as well. In a situation where Lyme disease is strongly suspected, such as in this child with erythema chronicum and a facial palsy, treatment is appropriate regardless of the serologic results.

A 13-year-old boy presents with a 3-week history of increasing left knee pain. He plays many sports at school, but does not remember any specific trauma. A radiograph is obtained.

1. Which of the following are the most likely physical examination findings?
   A. Pain with full flexion and a tender swollen mass in the posterior fossa
   B. Mild swelling and decreased, painful range of motion testing, with tenderness along the medial joint line
   C. No swelling and full passive range of motion, but tenderness at the tibial tubercle and pain with extension against force
   D. No swelling and full range of motion, but a positive patellar stress test
   E. No abnormality

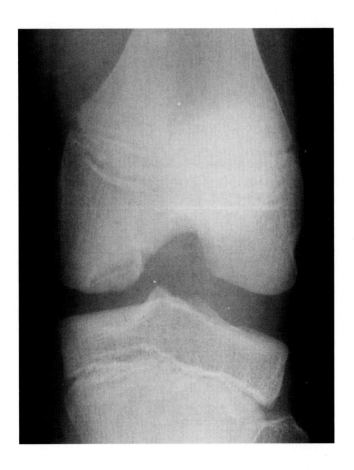

DISCUSSION

ANSWER:

1. E. No abnormality

1. You will find no abnormality, since the radiograph is consistent with osteochondritis dissecans. The findings in answer (A) are most consistent with a baker's cyst. These masses are either herniations of the synovium of the knee joint or a separate synovial cyst located in the popliteal fossa. Radiographs are usually normal or show the soft tissue swelling. The findings in answer (B) might be seen in a patient with a meniscal injury. These patients usually have a history of acute trauma initiating the knee pain and normal plain radiographs. The findings in answer (C) are most consistent with Osgood-Schlatter's disease. This disease is caused by chronic damage to the patellar tendon at its insertion into the tibial tuberosity during the child's growth spurt. The patient's pain is worsened by jumping or squatting which involve the quadriceps and patellar tendon. The tibial tuberosity is tender, may be swollen, and the patient may refuse or be unable to perform a deep knee bend. The radiograph is usually normal, but may show irregularity of the tibial tubercle. The findings in answer (D) are seen in patients with patellofemoral pain syndrome (PFPS), probably the most common cause of chronic knee pain in adolescents. PFPS is thought to be caused by malalignment of the extensor mechanism of the knee. The patients have chronic knee pain, especially when running and going down stairs. Their examination is usually normal except for the patellar stress test. To perform this test, the patient is placed in the supine position with the knee extended and relaxed. After you gently displace the patellar inferiorly, ask the patient to tighten the quadriceps or to "Push your knee into the bed" as you continue to press down on the patella. A patient with PFPS will have acute pain with this test. Radiographs will be normal.

Further Discussion

Osteochondritis dissecans is the separation of a small portion of the femoral condyle along with the overlying cartilage. Patients usually have a history of chronic pain related to activity. If the fragment is detached, the patient may have a history of momentary locking. If the pain is acutely associated with trauma, then an osteochondral fracture must be considered and an orthopedic surgeon consulted. In osteochondritis dissecans, the patient's examination is usually normal, although occasionally you can elicit some tenderness of the femoral condyle. The anteroposterior and lateral radiographs may be normal, and therefore a tunnel or intercondylar view should also be obtained for patients with chronic knee pain. These patients need careful follow-up since the prognosis is poor if the lesion has not healed before the growth plate closes.

A 5-year-old boy has a bleeding lesion of his forearm. According to his father, a "sore" first appeared 6 months ago and has enlarged. He thought it was just an abrasion when he first noted it, but now he is concerned that it has not resolved and that it frequently bleeds. The child is otherwise in good health. There is no history of malaise, weight loss, or bleeding gums. The general examination is normal. In particular, you do not appreciate any regional adenopathy, hepatosplenomegaly, or petechiae. The lesion on the forearm is 1 cm in diameter.

1. The diagnosis is:
   A. Hemangioma
   B. Molluscum contagiosum
   C. Malignant melanoma
   D. Pyogenic granuloma
   E. Neurofibroma

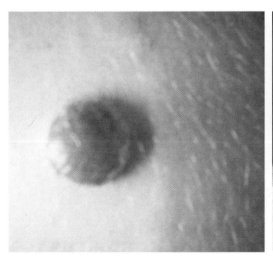 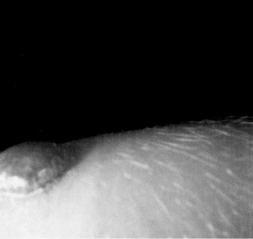

DISCUSSION

ANSWER:

1. D. Pyogenic granuloma

1. When confronted with a vascular lesion in childhood, the most likely diagnoses are hemangioma and pyogenic granuloma. This boy has a pyogenic granuloma. Since the lesion appeared well after the age of one year, it cannot be a hemangioma, as these are congenital or develop during the first 12 months of life. Neither neurofibromas nor molluscum are vascular in nature. While bleeding is a hallmark of malignant melanoma in adults, these cancerous lesions are exceeding rare in young children, unless a predisposing condition exists and the lesion contains pigment.

Further Discussion

Pyogenic granulomas occur frequently in children. Unfortunately the name provides no clue to the diagnosis, as the lesions are not pyogenic and do not contain granulomas on biopsy. Rather, they have a traumatic, not an infectious, origin, and consist of friable granulation tissue. The initiating event is usually trivial in nature, perhaps an insect bite or a small abrasion. For reasons that are not clear, the wound does not heal and the granulation tissue that forms in response to the injury proliferates. Each time the child sustains minor trauma to the area, local hemorrhage ensues. Generally, larger lesions, such as this one, require excision.

A 14-month-old is brought to the emergency department because of vomiting, lethargy, and foul-smelling stool. The mother presents the diaper shown below.

1. The most likely cause for this is:
   A. Iron ingestion
   B. Phenolphthalein ingestion
   C. Infection with Shigella
   D. Meckel's diverticulum
   E. Bowel obstruction

2. The most important diagnostic test to order is:
   A. Deferoxamine challenge
   B. Ferritin level
   C. Stool smear for white blood cells
   D. Barium enema
   E. Radionuclide scan

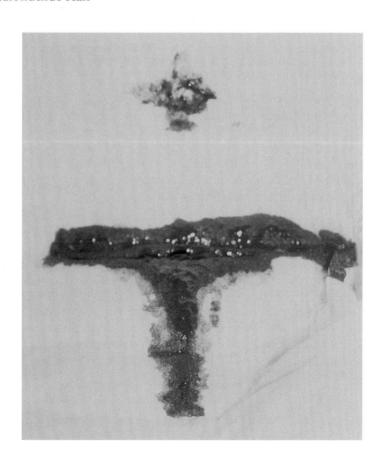

DISCUSSION

ANSWERS:
1. E. Bowel obstruction
2. D. Barium enema

1. This is a "currant jelly stool" that is characteristic of intussusception. It is a late finding in intussusception and is caused by the passage of a combination of blood and mucus. Intussusception occurs most commonly in the age range of 3-12 months, but may be seen throughout childhood. With this form of bowel obstruction, patients will have either recurrent colicky abdominal pain or periods of almost trance-like lethargy. Sometimes the painful phases and the lethargic periods will be intertwined. The other possible answers may all produce red or heme-positive stool; iron ingestion, hemolytic uremic syndrome and infection with Shigella may also cause central nervous system changes. Phenolphthalein is a dye that is used as a laxative, and thus may produce a red-colored diarrhea. Stool testing for blood should indicate that the stool is heme negative if this were the source. There would be no reason for the child having lethargy with this type of ingestion. Meckel's diverticulum may cause bright red, painless bleeding. The child's neurologic status should be normal and there should be no vomiting. A nuclear scan is the best way to establish the diagnosis.

   Iron poisoning produces bloody stools and a very protracted course of vomiting, as iron is a gastric irritant. The stools are usually a dark brown color from upper gastrointestinal bleeding. Shigella may produce bloody stools but usually in the context of profuse diarrhea and high fever. Often at this age, other family members are infected. Shigella toxin may produce seizures and irritability but usually not the characteristic lethargy seen with intussusception.

2. The best way to establish the diagnosis is through barium or air contrast enema. In equivocal cases, an abdominal ultrasound may give support to the diagnosis. If you suspect iron ingestion, then the best test to order is an abdominal radiograph to look for the opaque tablets. A Deferoxamine challenge test is reserved for those who are asymptomatic and have a negative radiograph, yet the diagnosis is still suspected. A stool smear for white blood studies is neither a sensitive nor specific test for establishing the diagnosis of Shigella infection.

Further Discussion

A "currant jelly stool" is found in about 60% of children with intussusception, but it is a relatively late occurrence. The most important step when intussusception is suspected is to arrange for a contrast enema. Both barium and air have been used to establish the diagnosis and treat the patient by reducing the intussusception. These procedures are successful in two-thirds of cases. Contraindications to attempting a contrast enema include signs of perforation, peritonitis or shock. These more advanced or complicated cases require surgical exploration and reduction. Most intussusception occurs spontaneously in the age group of the patient presented in this case. In children over 5-years-old, there may be an anatomical lead point found in over 75% of the cases.

CASE 42

A 15-month-old boy comes to the emergency department crying and refusing to move his arm after his father lifted him up by his hands and swung him around during play. He has a history of a previous fracture of the clavicle and his father gave him ibuprofen prior to arrival. Initially he refused to use the arm, but after returning from radiology with a radiograph, as shown, and with normal elbow and forearm radiographs, he actively uses the arm and has no deformity or tenderness.

1. Initial management would include:
   A. Obtaining an orthopedic consultation
   B. Casting his upper arm
   C. Applying a figure-of-eight splint
   D. Applying a sling and swath
   E. Instructions for the parents

2. What happened in radiology to make the child asymptomatic?
   A. The pain from his fractured clavicle decreased temporarily
   B. His nursemaid's elbow was reduced by the radiographer
   C. He became less anxious with the passage of time
   D. The arm pain decreased after administration of ibuprofen
   E. The displaced fracture of the clavicle was relocated

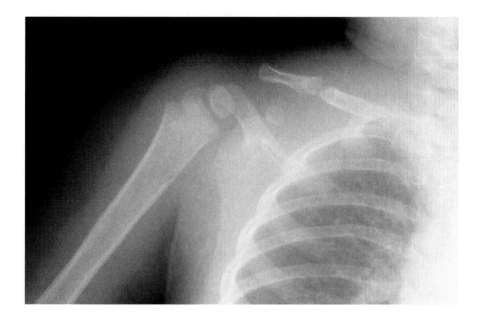

DISCUSSION

ANSWERS:
1. **E. Instructions for the parents**
2. **B. His nursemaid's elbow was reduced by the radiographer**

1. The child's radiograph shows a radiolucent area in the clavicle, with the contiguous clavicular ends cupped. This is a pseudoarthrosis of his right clavicle, not a fracture and does not need any specific therapy or consultations.

2. The patient's age, history of axial traction of a pronated and extended arm, nonfocal examination and spontaneous recovery in radiology makes the diagnosis of nursemaid's elbow likely. In children between 6 months and 5 years of age, the radial head subluxes during axial traction when the annular ligament becomes trapped in the radiohumeral joint. Various methods of reducing this injury have been recommended, usually involving supination of the wrist and either flexion or extension of the elbow. I personally recommend placing one hand over the child's elbow with one of your fingers over the radial head. Use your other hand to grasp the child's hand and quickly supinate the wrist and flex the elbow. If you have been successful, you will feel a "pop" over the radial head. Although the child may initially cry, within ten minutes the patient will be using the arm. During manipulation for elbow radiographs the patient's radial head may be reduced by the radiographer.

Further Discussion

Pseudoarthrosis of the clavicle is an unusual finding of uncertain pathogenesis. Some experts believe that the pseudoarthrosis represents a residual unhealed clavicular fracture acquired before or during the passage of the fetus through the birth canal. Interestingly, the lesions are almost always in the medial aspect of the right clavicle. Acquired lesions may be due to fractures that occurred after birth. Radiographs demonstrate a radiolucent area in the clavicle. The contiguous clavicular segments may be deformed and cupped or swollen.

A 14-year-old boy complains of chest pain over a 6-hour period. The pain began in the morning, when he was walking to school, and has persisted all day. Just a few minutes ago, while he was playing basketball in gym, the pain worsened. He describes it as a dull sensation, located substernally, with intermittent sharp twinges. His past medical history is remarkable for mild asthma, controlled with an albuterol inhaler, and a heart murmur.

Vital signs:	P 60/min R 18/min BP 130/85 mm Hg T 37.1°C
General:	Mildly obese, anxious, sweaty, no respiratory distress
Neck:	Supple, no jugular venous distension
Lungs:	Clear to auscultation and percussion
Heart:	Normal sinus rhythm, grade I/VI systolic ejection murmur; no gallops, rubs, or snaps
Chest:	Nontender
Abdomen:	No hepatosplenomegaly
Pulses:	4+ and symmetric in the upper and lower extremities

The nurse has obtained an EKG.

1. Your initial step is:
   A. Administer intravenous lidocaine
   B. Obtain an arterial blood gas
   C. Administer nebulized albuterol
   D. Consult cardiology
   E. None of the above

2. The most likely underlying cause for the pain is:
   A. Myocarditis
   B. Aortic aneurysm
   C. Pulmonary embolism
   D. Asthma
   E. None of the above

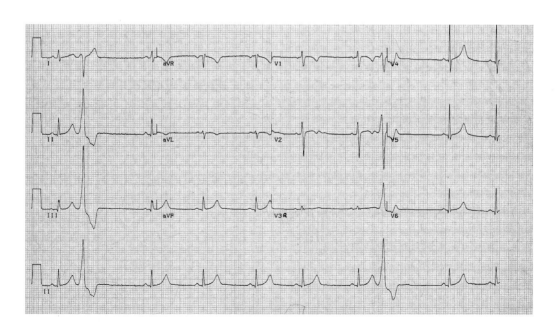

DISCUSSION

ANSWERS:
1. E. None of the above
2. E. None of the above

1 and 2. This teenager most likely has non specific chest pain. In the majority of children and adolescents with chest pain, no etiology is identified or the pain is presumed to be musculoskeletal, based on nondiagnostic physical findings. The EKG shows occasional, unifocal premature ventricular complexes. These complexes carry no clinical significance in this otherwise healthy child, who is hemodynamically stable. It is not surprising that this obese boy with chest pain all day is now anxious and sweaty after a game of basketball; one should not conclude that the cause is cardiac ischemia, which occurs during childhood and adolescence only in the face of several rare underlying conditions. Both aortic aneurysm and pulmonary embolism are distinctly uncommon, even in an obese teenager, and are unsupported by the history or physical examination. There is no hemoptysis, pleuritic or tearing pain, pleural rub, or diminished pulse in the lower extremities. No further studies or consultations are needed, although some might obtain a chest X-ray, perhaps to look for a small, spontaneous pneumothroax. Similarly, therapy would be limited to anti-inflammatory agents and/or reassurance.

Further Discussion

Both chest pain and premature ventricular contractions tend to evoke the specter of "heart" disease, particularly when they occur in combination. However, they are each common occurrences in otherwise healthy children and adolescents and, by chance, may be seen simultaneously. In particular, premature contractions affect a number of teenagers but only rarely portend trouble. One should have a higher level of concern in patients with any type of pre-existing cardiac disease or prior cardiac surgery, those with potentially cardiotoxic drugs circulating, and when the PVCs are other than isolated and unifocal.

Do children ever have myocardial infarctions? The answer is affirmative. Predisposing conditions include aberrant coronary arteries, aortic stenosis, Kawasaki disease, and certain inherited hyperlipidemias. In the presence of ischemia, one would expect to find ST segment and/or T wave abnormalities.

An 18-month-old girl comes to the emergency department with a rash. She was well until 12 hours earlier, when she developed a fever. After a call to the pediatrician, her mother treated her with acetaminophen. Her appetite has been decreased all day.

Vital signs:	P 180/min R 40/min BP 80/35 mm Hg T 39.2°C
General	Quiet, consolable
HEENT	Clear
Neck	Supple
Lungs	No rales
Heart	Sinus tachycardia, no murmurs or rubs
Abdomen	Nontender
Skin	A rash covers her whole body, as shown in the picture

You test the capillary refill on the dorsum of her foot by pressing with the thumb of your left hand and then picking up a camera and shooting this picture.

1. The most definite diagnostic test is:
   A. Blood culture
   B. Complete blood count
   C. Bone marrow aspiration
   D. Urinalysis
   E. Weil Felix titer

2. The treatment for this condition is:
   A. Intravenous gamma globulin
   B. Oral prednisone
   C. Intravenous cefotaxime
   D. Reassurance
   E. Oral tetracycline

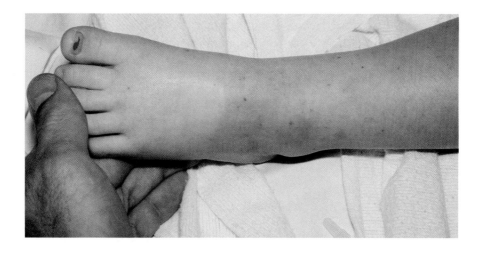

DISCUSSION

ANSWERS:
1. A. Blood culture
2. C. Intravenous cefotaxime

1. Given the sudden onset of fever followed a few hours later by a petechial rash in a child who has hypotension and delayed capillary refill, the diagnosis that jumps out at you is meningococcemia, which is the problem that brought this little girl to your attention. Thus, blood culture is the definite diagnostic test. One might see the organisms on a Gram stain of the cerebral spinal fluid; however, meningitis would not be likely in a case that progressed this rapidly, and her neck is supple. The second most likely diagnosis would be Rocky Mountain spotted fever (RMSF). Against this infection is the rapidity with which the rash and hemodynamic instability (hypotension, delayed capillary refill) followed on the heels of the fever. That's not to say that if this child presented during the summer in an area where RMSF was endemic, I might not hedge my bets and treat for both. Nevertheless, meningococcemia is far and away the most likely diagnosis here. The Weil-Felix test looks for antibodies against *Proteus*, which are sometimes elevated in RMSF, but the definitive test involves specific serology for antibodies to rickettsial antigens, usually performed by a reference laboratory. Could this be idiopathic thrombocytopenic purpura (ITP)? Not if you believe the capillary refill and are concerned about the blood pressure. For similar reasons, Henoch Schoenlein Purpura (HSP) seems unlikely; additionally, the rash of HSP usually has a more gradual onset and begins on the buttocks and lower extremities. A final diagnostic consideration might be a self-limited enteroviral infection. My advice is to err on the side of caution.

2. Cefotaxime provides excellent coverage for *Neisseria meningitidis* and other pathogens causing sepsis in previously healthy children, such as *Streptococcus pneumoniae* and the now rare *Haemophilus influenzae*. Prednisone and intravenous gamma globulin are used in ITP and the former agent has a role in selected cases of HSP. Usual therapies for RMSF include chloramphenicol and tetracycline. In a child this young and this ill, I would select the intravenous route.

Further Discussion

The use of capillary refill has both advocates and detractors. While the time for refill is influenced by environmental factors, a marked delay encountered in a child in a warm room strongly suggests poor perfusion to me. Additionally, one can monitor changes over time to assess the adequacy of therapy. Given the poor refill, in conjunction with tachycardia and hypotension, this child is profoundly ill. You can predict that her condition will deteriorate further with antibiotic treatment, presumably as a result of endotoxin release following bacterial killing. I would be inclined to place central venous and arterial catheters early in the course. Admission to the intensive care unit is appropriate.

This 15-year-old patient jammed his finger playing basketball.

1. A long term complication of this injury could result in:
   A. Boutonniere deformity
   B. Mallet finger
   C. Volkmann's contracture
   D. Tenosynovitis
   E. Myositis ossificans

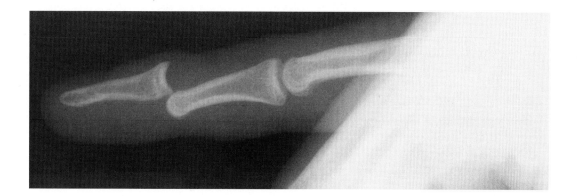

DISCUSSION

ANSWER:

1. **B. Mallet finger**

1. The boutonniere deformity occurs after a proximal interphalangeal dislocation. During this injury the central slip of the extensor tendon may be torn and the lateral bands of the extensor mechanism may then drop anteriorly. The joint has now "buttonholed" through the lateral bands. The patient cannot fully extend the proximal interphalangeal (PIP) joint. If this is blamed on pain and the dislocation is not recognized, appropriately splinted and referred, a boutonniere deformity may result. In this deformity the metacarpophalangeal joint and distal interphalangeal (DIP) joint are extended and the PIP flexed. Volkmann's ischemic contracture results as a complication of supracondylar fractures leading to compromise of blood flow around the elbow. Infectious tenosynovitis is not usually seen after closed finger injuries. Myositis ossificans can develop whenever a muscle has a hematoma, but is more commonly seen after quadriceps contusion or an elbow dislocation. This patient's injury, a DIP dislocation, may result in a mallet, or baseball finger, if the extensor tendon is avulsed and not treated appropriately. A mallet finger is held in continuous flexion as the flexor tendons are unopposed by the avulsed extensor tendon.

Further Discussion

For all dislocations, it is important to obtain at least two views of the affected joint. The PIP joint is usually easily reduced after anesthesia with a digital block. Wrap the involved finger with gauze to facilitate your grip and then reduce the dislocation with in-line traction. It may help to hyperextend the joint, increasing the deformity, prior to pushing the phalanx back into position along with the in-line traction. If unsuccessful, do not blame your technique and continue multiple attempts at reduction. The joint may not reduce because of soft tissue interposing in the joint space, and open reduction by an orthopedic surgeon may be required. Post-reduction care consists of splinting the DIP in extension while allowing full range of motion of the PIP for 3 weeks and referral to an orthopedic surgeon.

CASE 46

A 6-year-old girl is brought to the emergency department for a fever and cough. Her temperature is 39.5°C, pulse 100/min, respirations 30/min, and BP 120/96 mm Hg. The examination of her HEENT is positive for a left ear infection and a red pharynx. An abnormality of the skin is noted, confined to the area of the chest.

1. Based on your findings you would:
    A. File a child abuse report
    B. Evaluate the child for a bleeding disorder
    C. Diagnose herpes zoster and start acyclovir
    D. Start intravenous ceftriaxone
    E. None of the above

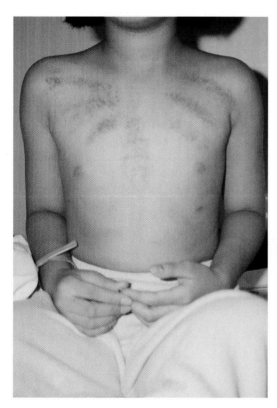
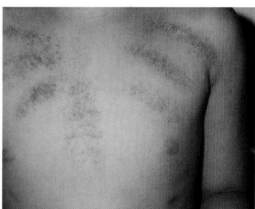

DISCUSSION

ANSWER:

1. **E. None of the above**

1. This is a classic example of coining or *cao gio,* a folk remedy used in Southeast Asia to treat respiratory infections. The edge of the coin is used to abrade the skin along the rib margins and sternum. The raw skin presumably allows the infectious elements to leave the body. A similar technique is common in China. It is performed with the edge of a spoon and is called *Quat sha.* The concern about herpetic infection and treatment with acyclovir should be eliminated when examining the skin closely and not finding any vesicles; additionally, the eruption is bilateral and nondermatomal. Although a close examination of the skin will reveal petechial lesions caused by the trauma of abrasion, these should not be mistaken for the lesions of a vasculitis or bleeding diathesis. Your next move here is amoxicillin for the otitis media, followed by discharge home.

Further Discussion

If you have not seen coining, it is a very striking finding. The geometric pattern suggests, even to the inexperienced observer, some sort of mechanical trauma. Unfortunately, this explanation is often equated with child abuse, which it is not.

A 16-year-old young man complains only that he has had an enlarging lesion on his penis for 3 weeks. He has not experienced any malaise or fever. His past medical history is notable for recurrent streptococcal pharyngitis and anemia. On examination, he is well appearing and afebrile. His neck is supple with shoddy adenopathy bilaterally. The lungs are clear to auscultation, and there are no cardiac murmurs. He has no hepatosplenomegaly or abdominal tenderness.

Several 1 × 2 cm nontender lymph nodes are palatable in the left inguinal area, and a single 1 × 1 cm lymph node is felt on the right.

1. The most likely diagnosis is
   A. Chancroid
   B. Lymphogranuloma venereum
   C. Herpes simplex
   D. Syphilis
   E. Condyloma acuminata

2. The appropriate treatment is:
   A. Intramuscular procaine penicillin
   B. Oral cefixime
   C. Intramuscular ceftriaxone
   D. Intravenous penicillin G
   E. None of the above

3. Which of the following tests would you do?
   A. HIV titer
   B. Urethral swab for gonorrhea
   C. RPR
   D. Darkfield examination
   E. All of the above

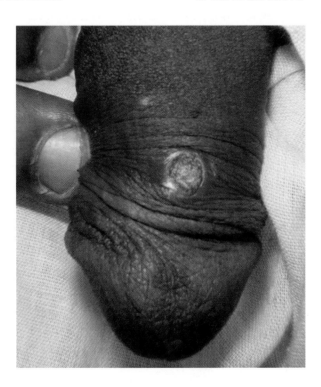

DISCUSSION

ANSWERS:
1. D. Syphilis
2. E. None of the above
3. E. All of the above

1. The patient has a chancer of primary syphilis, but I will offer half credit for chancroid. Lymphogranuloma venereum causes enlargement of the inguinal lymph nodes bilaterally (to a much greater degree than in this patient), but not an ulcer. Vesicles are characteristic of Herpes simplex and the duration in this case is longer than the usual 2 weeks. While chancroid is a possibility, it is less common in the United States than syphilis and is usually painful; this boy complained only of a lesion and not pain. Condyloma acuminata form pedunculated lesions.

2. None of the treatments listed are appropriate, as benzathine penicillin is recommended for syphilis. In primary disease, a single injection of 2.4 million units suffices. Procaine penicillin, formerly a first line therapy for gonorrhea, successfully eradicates incubating syphilis (in patients with no lesions and negative serology), but it will not treat established disease. Intravenous penicillin is the proper choice for neurosyphilis. Cefixime and ceftriaxone have a role for gonorrhea rather than syphilis.

3. Get all of the above. Birds of a feather flock together, and this patient is at risk for having multiple sexually transmitted diseases (STDs). A darkfield examination and RPR test for syphilis, a swab of the urethra is appropriate for gonorrhea (not treated by benzathine penicillin), and the CDC recommends testing for HIV when another STD is present. Either one of or both the darkfield examination or the RPR may be positive; occasionally, both will be negative. The darkfield examination identifies spirochetes in the exudate of the ulcer and is reasonably sensitive in skilled hands. The RPR is a serologic test that is highly reliable, once antibodies have formed. Since the chancer occurs 4-8 weeks after infection and the antibodies arise after 6-12 weeks, the darkfield examination may be negative or positive and the RPR negative early on; with time, both should be positive, but the spirochetes are not always seen on darkfield examination.

Further Discussion

Syphilis is common, although much less so in the pediatric than in the adult population. A recent surge in the incidence has been tied to the epidemic of crack cocaine, with young women trading sex for money. Thus, we are seeing two populations with this disease, teenagers who have acquired the infection through sexual activity and infants who are infected congenitally.

An 8-year-old is brought in for a skin rash. Her mother states that the eruption started as a mosquito bite. Your examination shows the following:

1. Based on this finding you would:
   A. Treat the child with oral cephalexin
   B. Treat with oral acyclovir
   C. Treat with IV ceftriaxone
   D. Apply topical corticosteroids
   E. Apply DEET

2. The most likely complication despite treatment that this child might incur is:
   A. Toxic shock syndrome
   B. Acute glomerulonephritis
   C. Acute rheumatic fever
   D. Encephalitis
   E. Eczema herpeticum

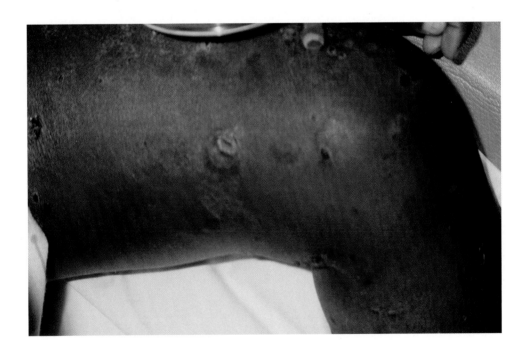

DISCUSSION

ANSWERS:
1. A. Treat the child with oral cephalexin
2. B. Acute gomerulonephritis

1. The findings are of impetigo, which may be treated with oral cephalexin. The parent's report of an insect bite that is scratched and inoculated with streptococci is a typical history. Acyclovir is not indicated, as the lesions do not appear to be herpetic, in that they are too large, do not have a red base, and do not appear to be vesicular. Herpetic lesions may be difficult to diagnose by appearance alone and if there is any question, a Tzanck preparation will show the presence of multinucleated giant cells. Using ceftriaxone would be effective, but this represents overkill and should be reserved for more serious infections. Topical corticosteroids are appropriate for atopic or contact dermatitis, and DEET is administered prophylactically as an insect repellant.

2. There are likely to be no complications. Of those listed, acute post-streptococcal glomerulonephritis is the most common. Streptococcal and staphylococcal toxic shock syndromes do not usually follow a treated superficial skin infection. Rheumatic fever also does not occur after a skin infection.

Further Discussion

Impetigo is generally a problem in warm, humid climates. In the past, two types were identified. In some cases of impetigo, there were crusted scabbed lesions. These were often due to streptococci. Other cases were noted to have a bullous nature, and these were attributed to staphylococci. These distinctions have now broken down, and some of the honey colored crusted lesion may be caused by staphylococci. Thus, there is a need for broader coverage than simple penicillin. An alternative strategy would be to start with penicillin and, if the lesions were continuing to spread, to switch to an anti-staphylococcal agent.

CASE 49

A 12-year-old male presents to the emergency department after becoming upset at school, turning pale, losing consciousness, and falling to the floor. He regained consciousness after about 1 minute, and has been fine since. His teacher says that the patient has fainted in class before. His EKG tracing is below.

1. In addition to an EKG this patient also needs the following test:
   A. Complete blood count (CBC)
   B. Lipid levels
   C. Full toxicology screen
   D. Glucose level
   E. None of the above

2. If the above test is unrevealing, then therapy of this patient's likely disorder may include:
   A. Beta adrenergic blocking agents.
   B. Cardiovascular fitness training
   C. Mineralocorticoids.
   D. Atropine
   E. Potassium

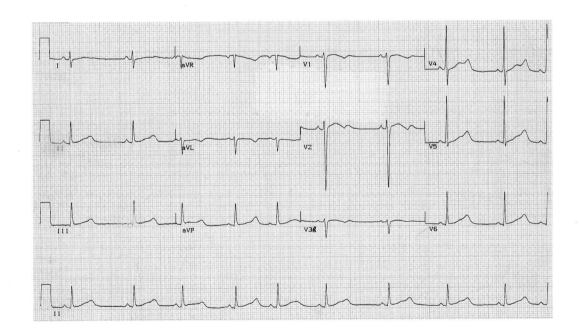

DISCUSSION

ANSWERS:

1. C. Full toxicology screen
2. A. Beta adrenergic blocking agents

1. Although severe anemia and hypoglycemia may cause syncope, the EKG findings in this patient make these tests unlikely to be helpful (a CBC and glucose level should often be obtained in patients with a history of syncope). Lipid levels may be associated with increased risks of coronary artery disease in this patient's future, but are unlikely to be worthwhile emergently. Given the finding on this EKG, an immediate full toxicology screen should be obtained.

2. The EKG tracing shows sinus bradycardia, an extremely prolonged QTc (about 560 ms), bizarre T waves, and a sinus arrhythmia. Syncope and a prolonged QTc interval can be caused by various drugs, such as tricyclic antidepressants, phenothiazines, and antiarrhythmic agents, hypocalcemia, or myocarditis. If the patient's toxicology screen and calcium level are unrevealing, and the patient has no signs of myocarditis, then the most likely diagnosis is one of the congenital prolonged QTc syndromes, such as Romano-Ward. Many experts suggest beta adrenergic agents to decrease sympathetic activity of the heart and the risk of sudden death. Cardiovascular fitness training is not routinely recommended. Severe recurrent vasodepressor syncope is occasionally treated by cardiologists with mineralocorticoids. Patients with asymptomatic bradycardia should not be treated with atropine. Standard guidelines advocate for atropine only when the bradycardia is associated with serious symptoms (e.g., chest pain or shortness of breath) or signs (e.g., hypotension, shock, pulmonary congestion, congestive heart failure, or acute myocardial infarction).

Further Discussion

This patient's extremely prolonged QTc makes a congenital prolonged QTc syndrome very likely. Because the Jervell and Lange-Nielsen syndromes are associated with congenital deafness, Romano-Ward, an autosomal dominant syndrome with normal hearing, becomes more likely. Patients usually present with recurrent syncope, often precipitated by loud noises or emotions. The episodes may be mistaken for neurologic events like breath holding or seizures, delaying the diagnosis. Once a patient is identified with QTc prolongation, an EKG should be obtained in all family members. The inherited defect involves a membrane protein regulating potassium flux across the myocyte. These patients are at high risk for ventricular arrhythmias including torsade de pointes and sudden death. Therapy consists of prophylactic beta-blockers. If pharmacological therapy is unsuccessful, pacing, left cervicothoracic sympathectomy, or an implantable automatic defibrillator may be necessary.

A 14-month-old boy arrives in status epilepticus, following a febrile illness that began the preceding day. The parents are poor historians and do not offer much history. After two doses of intravenous lorazepam, his seizures stop but he remains obtunded. He strikes you as small for his age. His temperature is 38.2°C. You note that his pupils are 2 mm, equal, and reactive, but you cannot visualize the fundi. His neck is supple. Several bruises are notable over the anterior tibia. You obtain a portable chest X-ray (normal cardiac silhouette, no infiltrates) and a skeletal survey. While you await the results of laboratory assays, he begins to convulse again:

1. Your next step is:
   A. CT scan of the head
   B. Intravenous fosphenytoin
   C. Intravenous calcium
   D. Neurosurgical consultation
   E. Intravenous ceftriaxone

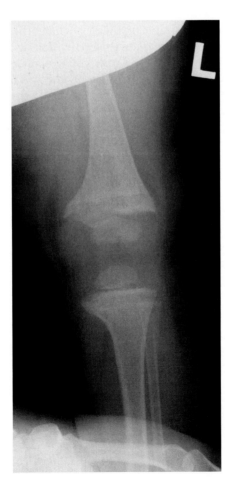

DISCUSSION

ANSWER:

1. **C. Intravenous calcium**

1. As the boy has rickets, you treat with intravenous calcium, anticipating hypocalcemia that is confirmed minutes later with a level of 5.3 mg/dl. Child abuse causing subarachnoid hemorrhage is in the differential diagnosis for seizures in infancy. Generally, one would start the evaluation for any type of cerebral injury with a CT scan of the head and obtain an immediate neurosurgical consultation only if concerned about an expanding intracranial lesion, requiring urgent evacuation. Symmetric, reactive pupils and the absence of focal neurologic findings weigh against acute herniation. Given the presence of fever followed by seizures, meningitis is high up on the list of causes. The lack of nuchal rigidity is inconsequential in a patient who is postictal. While I commend those readers who chose to give ceftriaxone (and I would do the same), it will not stop the seizures even in the face of a central nervous system infection. A more appropriate response is calcium, once you have seen the X-ray. Similarly, it would not be incorrect to administer fosphenytoin, which might stop the seizures as did the lorazepam, but it is not the best approach here.

Further Discussion

While debates continue as to the appropriate extent of the evaluation for seizures, these arguments usually apply to either simple febrile or brief afebrile convulsions. Status epilepticus, on the other hand, is a life-threatening emergency that demands a thorough work-up. Thus, even if you did not obtain long bone X-rays, you would have discovered the decreased serum calcium in short order. Hypocalcemia may be artifactual in patients with hypoproteinemia or result from disorders such as hypoparathyroidism and rickets. The varieties of rickets include primary vitamin D deficiency, secondary vitamin D deficiency (malabsorption, chronic renal failure), or vitamin D resistance at the level of the end organ receptor. None of these entities are common, but vitamin D deficiency is seen frequently among inner city children in certain religious sects that engage in the combination of swaddling and prolonged breast feeding. Several small epidemics have been described in the past few years.

A 6-week-old infant is brought to the hospital by both his parents at 2:00 AM because he has been crying incessantly. At noon on the previous day, he was seen by a physician who diagnosed colic and treated him with simethicone. When his crying persisted, his parents brought him to the emergency department after dinner. The parents were told that fluorescein staining of his cornea was negative but were given ophthalmic ointment in case he had a small corneal abrasion. Nothing has worked. You are frustrated to find no abnormalities on examination until you remove the socks.

1. The cause of this condition is a:
   A. Foreign body
   B. Congenital lesion
   C. Infectious disease
   D. Social problem
   E. Vascular anomaly

2. Your treatment includes:
   A. Surgical intervention
   B. Topical antibiotics
   C. Filing an abuse report
   D. Systemic antibiotics
   E. None of the above

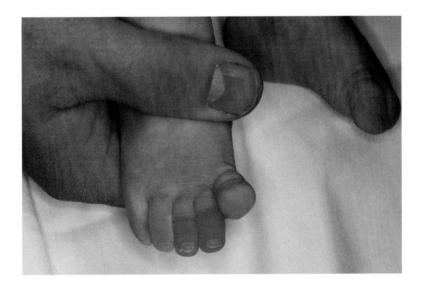

DISCUSSION

ANSWERS:

1. **A. Foreign body**
2. **A. Surgical intervention**

1. This child has a foreign body, in this case a hair, wrapped around two of his toes. It is an accidental injury.

2. Treatment involves removal of the offending hair in the emergency department. Sometimes the end is visible and can be use to unwind the hair. More often, one must explore the wound and dissect out the strands. While older texts may refer to the use of depilatories, they are not recommended, since they are ineffective and irritating.

Further Discussion

Hair-tourniquet syndrome is a relatively frequent occurrence that can involve the fingers, toes, penis, or clitoris. It is an easy diagnosis to make if you think of it and undertake a diligent search. As an encircling hair dries out, it shrinks, cuts through the skin, and sinks below the surface. Thus, a cursory look at the digits and other appendages may fail to identify the culprit. Of course, once you make the diagnosis, treatment is easy. NOT!! One or more hairs may be wrapped around one or more times, occasionally almost at the level of the phalanx, when the digit is involved. A meticulous hunt for every last strand is essential. Even using my loupes, on occasion I have been unable to convince myself that I have removed every vestige of hair and have referred patients for exploration in the operating suite.

The textbooks claim that one of this child's parents is likely to have long hair of a particular color. For bonus points, which color?

An almost 13-year-old girl complains that she started to "pass out" at school. She awoke that morning feeling nauseous and seemed "weak" all day. In response to your specific question, she states that she has lost 20 pounds over the past 3 months, which she attributes to a deliberate attempt to lose weight in preparation for buying a new dress for an upcoming celebration. Her pediatrician counseled her not to continue dieting, but she has ignored this advice. On examination, she appears thin but in no acute distress. She is afebrile with a pulse of 110/min and respirations of 18/min. Her blood pressure is 95/55 mm Hg lying down and 80/35 mm Hg standing.

1. You anticipate the following laboratory results:
   A. Serum glucose 600 mg/dl and urine ketones 4+
   B. Serum glucose 400 mg/dl and serum Na 125 mEq/L
   C. Serum potassium 2.5 mEq/L and serum Na 125 mEq/L
   D. Serum glucose 50 mg/dl and serum K 2.5 mEq/L
   E. Serum glucose 50 mEq/L and serum Na 125 mEq/L

2. Other possible findings might include:
   A. An EKG with U waves
   B. Splenomegaly
   C. A history of sexual abuse
   D. A CBC with eosinophilia
   E. Midline neck swelling

3. After a bolus of normal saline, you recommend treatment with:
   A. Methylprednisolone
   B. Dietary therapy
   C. Methimazole
   D. Thyroid hormone
   E. Insulin

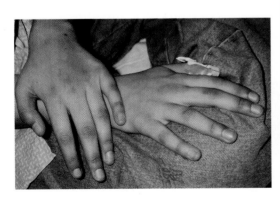
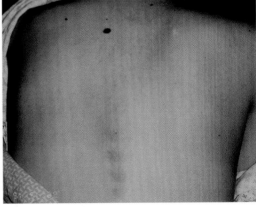

DISCUSSION

ANSWERS:
1. E. Serum glucose 50 mEq/L and serum Na 125 mEq/L
2. D. A CBC with eosinophilia
3. A. Methylprednisolone

1. This preteenager has Addison's disease or adrenal failure that leads to a deficiency of both mineralocorticoids and glucocorticoids. Thus, expected laboratory abnormalities include hypoglycemia, hyponatremia, and hyperkalemia; the most likely findings are a glucose of 50 mg/dl and a Na of 125 mEq/L. Diabetes mellitus causes hyperglycemia and ketonuria; additionally, either hypo- or hyperkalemia may occur. Patients with anorexia nervosa vomit frequently and may develop hypokalemia.

2. An additional finding in some patients with Addison's disease is eosinophilia, which may also occur with neoplasms, allergic disorders, collagen vascular diseases, and parasitic infestations. U waves on the EKG, a sign of hypokalemia, could be seen with anorexia nervosa or diabetes mellitus. A midline neck swelling, or goiter, would suggest thyroiditis or Grave's disease. A history of sexual abuse is uncovered more often in females with eating disorders than in the general population. Splenomegaly occurs in approximately 60% of teens and young adults with infectious mononucleosis.

3. After the saline bolus, the next most urgent therapy for Addison's disease is glucocorticoid therapy. Mineralocorticoid administration can be delayed as long as other measures (saline infusion) are taken to correct hyponatremia and hyperkalemia. Insulin is appropriate for diabetes mellitus, which is often accompanied by a history of weight loss for 2 to 3 weeks rather than 2 to 3 months. Thyroid hormone is appropriate for hypothyroidism, and methimazole for Grave's disease. Except in cases of thyroid storm or myxedema coma, specific treatment for abnormal thyroid function should await confirmatory results from the laboratory.

Further Discussion

This nearly 13-year-old girl with a history of several months of weight loss developed syncope and is noted to have hyperpigmentation, making Addison's disease the likely diagnosis. While she is just a bit on the young side, the story without the cutaneous findings fits well with anorexia nervosa. I have seen several teenage girls receive therapy for presumed anorexia nervosa, who subsequently presented with syncope, hyponatremia, and hyperpigmentation, leading to the correct diagnosis of adrenal failure.

A father complains that his 3-week-old infant cries all the time. According to him, the child has been "colicky" since birth, but the situation has gotten worse over the last 2 days. He has been giving the infant paregoric, which was prescribed for the crying at his check up 1 week ago. The infant was born after a 37-week gestation, weighing 5 lb, 12 oz. Pregnancy was complicated by maternal hypertension and proteinuria.

Vital signs:	P 134/min R 28/min BP 92/56 mm Hg T 37.4°C
General	Uncomfortable, more irritable when held
Head	Anterior fontanel flat
Eyes	No conjunctivitis
Ears	Tympanic membranes pearly gray
Nodes	No adenopathy
Neck	Supple
Lungs	No rales or wheezes
Heart	No murmurs
Abdomen	Mild tenderness; liver palpable 2 cm below the right costal margin
Neurologic	Lethargic with no focal findings

1. Your diagnosis is:
   A. Incarcerated hernia
   B. Septic arthritis
   C. Intussusception
   D. Infantile colic
   E. Pelvic fracture

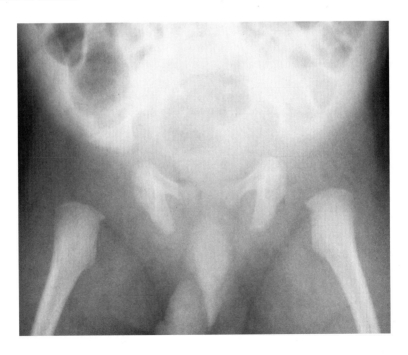

DISCUSSION

ANSWER:

1. B. Septic arthritis

1. The X-ray shows a dislocated right hip. While the most common cause of this problem is congenital dislocation, this disorder is painless and does not cause any symptoms. In the setting of a persistently crying infant with paradoxical irritability, the focus switches to septic arthritis. Infection in the hip joint can dislocate the hip, as pus under pressure stretches the capsule and supporting structures, which are relatively weak at this point in life. The pelvic bones are normal for age. While both incarcerated hernia and intussusception stand high on the list in the differential diagnosis for the crying infant, the limited view of the viscera on this X-ray shows no abnormality.

Further Discussion

The differential diagnosis of the "crying infant" is extensive. Life threatening conditions that must be considered include meningitis, intussusception, and incarcerated hernia. Other disorders that cause persistent pain are corneal abrasion, otitis media, septic arthritis/ osteomyelitis, and hair tourniquet syndrome. On the other hand, the most frequent reason for crying is infantile colic, defined as excessive crying occurring in children 3 weeks to 3 months of age. In the acute care setting, one most be wary of presuming that the problem is colic, which should be a diagnosis of exclusion. A thorough examination of every region of the body is mandatory. Even when negative, the physician should be cautious about telling the parents that the problem is colic and should instead simply state, at the time of the first acute care visit, that no evidence of an emergent cause for the crying has been found, but that follow up is necessary. A careful approach is particularly important for the infant who cries persistently during the visit; cessation of crying is somewhat reassuring, as most of the serious disorders do not wax and wane.

Staphylococcus aureus is the most common etiology for septic hip, but in the newborn period Group B streptococci are important pathogens and *Hemophilus influenzae* may be seen in unvaccinated children, primarily between 3 months and 3 years of age. Once this condition is suspected, time is of the essence, as pus under pressure may compromise the blood supply to the femoral head. Following aspiration of the joint to confirm the diagnosis, treatment consists of open drainage.

An 8-month-old child developed a lesion 3 days ago, which has increased in size. Her mother reports that she has had no fever or decrease in appetite, but has been fussier than usual. Past medical history is remarkable for a 36-week gestation with a birth weight of 2.6 kg and one admission for bronchiolitis at age 5 months. The family lives on a farm in Vermont and denies recent travel.

Vital signs	P 130/min R 24/min BP 95/55 mm Hg T 37.8°C
General	Fussy but consolable
HEENT	Clear
Lungs	No rales
Heart	Sinus tachycardia, no murmurs or rubs
Abdomen	Nontender, no hepatomegaly, spleen palpable 1 cm below the right costal margin
Extremities	Full range of motion

1. The most likely cause of this supraclavicular lesion is:
   A. *Mycobacterium tuberculosis*
   B. *Streptococcus pyogenes*
   C. *Bartonella hensleae*
   D. *Staphylococcus aureus*
   E. *Mycobacterium*

2. Treatment is:
   A. Incision
   B. Erythromycin
   C. Ceftriaxone
   D. Amoxicillin-clavulanate
   E. Excision

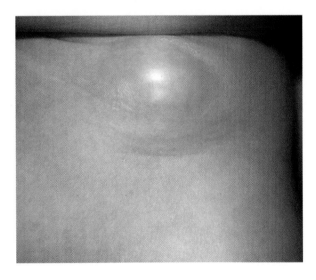

DISCUSSION

ANSWERS:

1. D. *Staphylococcus aureus*
2. A. Incision

1. This child has a mass in his supraclavicular fossa. In adults, a lesion in this area raises the possibility of a lymphoma or a metastatic gastric carcinoma (sentinel node of Virchow). Although neoplastic disease is less common in children, nodes in the supraclavicular area are more concerning than those in the neck, axilla, or groin. However, in this child, the clinical examination reveals an obviously shiny, tense, fluctuant node that screams "infection" at you. In order, the likely causes for a solitary infected lymph node are pyogenic bacteria, *Bartonella hensleae* (cat scratch disease), a number of atypical mycobacteria (scrofula), and very rarely without a travel history, tuberculosis. Over 90% of cases result from pyogenic bacterial infections; of these, the most common is *S. aureus*, followed by *S. pyogenes* (Group A beta-hemolytic *Streptococcus*).

2. Successful treatment by incision and drainage is illustrated. Once a lymph node develops fluctuance, antibiotic therapy alone, with any drug by any route, will not do the trick. An alternative approach in an otherwise healthy, afebrile, well-appearing child is to aspirate the purulent material and begin oral antibiotics. The patient then returns daily and a repeat aspiration is undertaken if pus reaccumulates. Excision is not indicated for a fluctuant node of brief duration.

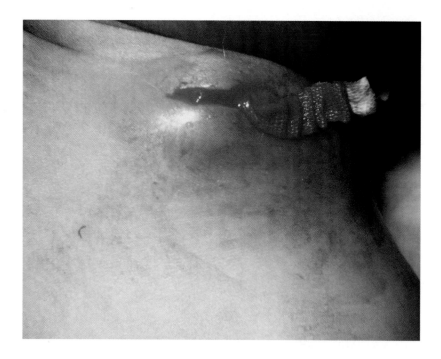

This 5-year-old had been febrile for the last 24 hours and is refusing to drink. With the exception of his tongue, the rest of his examination is normal.

His symptoms are caused by:

A. Behçet's disease
B. Aphthous stomatitis
C. Herpetic stomatitis
D. Hand, Foot, Mouth disease
E. Vincent's angina or trench mouth

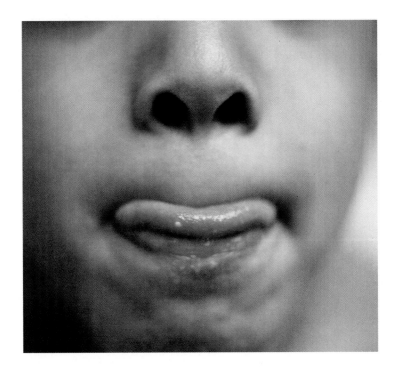

DISCUSSION

ANSWER:

1. **C. Herpetic stomatitis**

1. This child has herpetic stomatitis, usually due to Herpes simplex virus type 1. This is a very common infection from infancy through the early school years. The lesions begin as vesicles but may ulcerate and may involve the tongue (stomatitis), gingiva (gingivitis), and lips (labiitis). This child's infection is mild and early in its course. These lesions may progress to erythematous ulcerations and hemorrhage and may even involve the perioral skin. Fever and cervical lymphadenopathy are common. Behçet's disease is a rare disorder in adults and extremely rare in school-age children. The patients have oral ulcers along with conjunctivitis or iritis and genital ulcerations. This patient appears to have pustules or vesicles on his tongue without ulcerations. Aphthous stomatitis or canker sores may begin as focal areas of painful erythema, but soon progress to shallow gray white erosions or ulcers. Hand, Foot, Mouth disease is a viral infection, caused by Coxsackie A16, and presents with fever and oral vesicles. The oral lesions of Coxsackie infection are usually in the posterior pharynx and not on the tongue. In addition, flat, often elliptical lesions with surrounding erythema on the fingers, toes, palms, and soles are seen. Vincent's angina or trench mouth is more frequently seen in adolescents. This disorder mainly affects the gingiva, especially the gingival margins, which are painful, swollen, ulcerated, and often hemorrhagic. The gingival papillae, normally seen between the teeth, are missing or "punched out" in this infection.

Further Discussion

The most common complication is dehydration due to refusal to drink. Systemic analgesics (e.g., acetaminophen, ibuprofen or codeine) and topical analgesics (e.g., 2% viscous xylocaine rinses or a 1:1 mixture of diphenhydramine and Kaopectate) may help the child drink. Oral acyclovir has not been shown to be effective in nonimmunosuppressed patients.

Worried parents bring their 2-year-old girl to the emergency department because she is "very sick." A recent immigrant to the United States, she has been previously healthy, but this afternoon she became lethargic, vomited once, and held her abdomen "in pain." Now her parents feel that she seems to be very pale and is breathing rapidly. Your initial examination shows an ill-appearing child with a rectal temperature of 37.2°C, a pulse of 175/min, a respiratory rate of 44/min, and blood pressure of 78/46 mm Hg. The two photographs demonstrate her abdominal and skin examination.

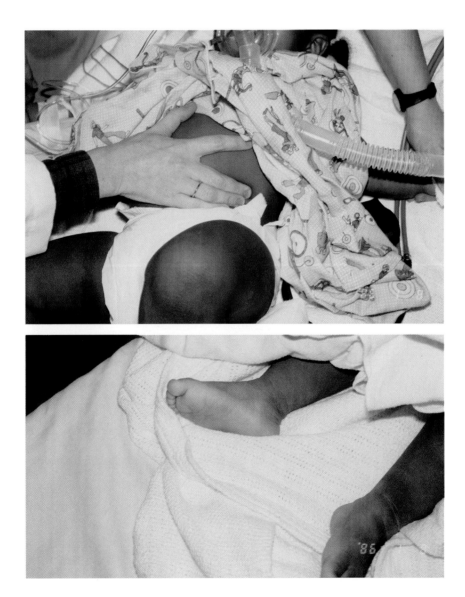

1. You immediately assess her airway and obtain vascular access. The therapy for this patient's life-threatening condition requires:
   A. Surgical consultation
   B. Intravenous ceftriaxone
   C. Dopamine infusion
   D. Blood transfusion
   E. Plasmapheresis

DISCUSSION

ANSWER:
1. **D. Blood transfusion**

1. The sudden presentation of an acutely ill child with no obvious diagnosis is always an anxiety provoking experience. Her ill appearance and abnormal vital signs suggest that she is in shock, but why? The two photographs show that she is an African American, and that she has an enlarged spleen and pale skin.

    Patients with surgical emergencies can present in shock from conditions such as a ruptured appendix or an intestinal perforation, due to child abuse or unwitnessed trauma. Additionally, many infectious disease emergencies, such as meningitis, sepsis, and toxic shock syndrome may manifest with signs of shock, as may certain oncologic emergencies, such as acute leukemia or aplastic anemia. However, an afebrile, pale, African American child with splenomegaly is most likely ill due to acute splenic sequestration, for which the initial therapy is an immediate transfusion of 10 to 20 cc/kg of packed RBCs or whole blood.

Further Discussion

Acute splenic sequestration is one of the life-threatening complications of sickle cell disease in young children; sequestration can occur as well in older patients with sickle beta thalassemia or sickle hemoglobin C disease. 20% of patients with sickle cell disease present with sequestration as the first manifestation of their disease. Other common presenting manifestations include dactylitis, pneumococcal infection and painful crises. Patients under 2-years-old, whose spleens are not yet fibrotic but are still distensible, are most susceptible to acute splenic sequestration, although about 20% of these crises occur between 2 and 6 years of age. The sickled cells obstruct splenic outflow leading to massive enlargement of the spleen with a large proportion of the circulating blood volume. This results in hypovolemic shock and often death, if it is not promptly recognized and treated. The diagnosis should be suspected in any African American child presenting with pallor, splenomegaly and shock. The laboratory findings of a decreased (from baseline) hematocrit and higher than usual reticulocyte count confirm the diagnosis. Occasionally crystalloid volume expansion may cause the spleen to "release" enough nonsickled red blood cells to reverse the shock, but usually a transfusion of 10 to 20 cc/kg of packed RBC or whole blood is required. Splenectomy is a consideration in any patient who has had one or more of these acutely life-threatening events.

A 14-year-old girl comes to the emergency department due to a 3-day history of a swollen, painful eye.

1. Initial therapy should consist of:
    A. Incision and drainage
    B. Cephalexin
    C. Warm compresses
    D. Surgical excision
    E. Aspiration

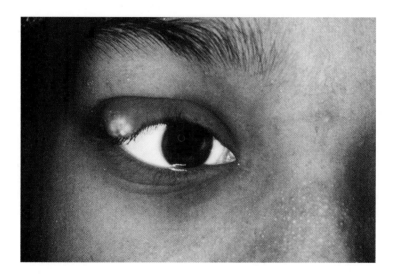

DISCUSSION

ANSWERS:

1. C. **Warm compresses**

1. Masses on the eyelid may be due to internal or external (stye) hordeolum, chalazions, or tumors. If the glands of the lid are acutely infected, the mass is tender, red, and may have a white pustular center as in this case. If the glands of Zeis, adjacent to the eyelid follicle, are involved, the abscess points at the lid margin. This is termed an external hordeolum or stye. If the meibomian glands, within the tarsal plate, are involved, the abscess may point out through the skin, as in this patient, or inward to the conjunctival surface. This is called an internal hordeolum. For this abscess, the first line of therapy is frequent warm compresses. The stye will usually open, drain and resolve. Aspiration will not hasten the resolution. If compresses fail, incision and drainage may be necessary. If untreated, the abscess may spread to adjacent tissues causing cellulitis, which would then require oral antimicrobials, such as cephalexin. The meibomian glands can also develop into a chronic granulomatous mass, a chalazion, without signs of acute inflammation. The chalazion may require surgical excision if it distorts vision or causes a cosmetic problem. Except for hemangiomas, tumors of the eyelids are rare. Malignant tumors, such as basal cell and squamous cell carcinoma, are extremely rare and have abnormal overlying epithelium.

A 3-month-old infant arrives in the emergency department in acute distress. Her pulse is 190/min, respiration is 40/min, and her termperature is 35.9°C rectally, her blood pressure is undetectable. Several attempts at peripheral intravenous access are unsuccessful, but an intraosseous needle and a central venous catheter are placed.

1. This catheter was placed by directing a needle:
   A. Under the junction of the proximal and middle thirds of the clavicle toward the sternal notch
   B. At the apex of the junction of the two heads of the sternocleidomastoid toward the contralateral nipple
   C. Under the junction of the proximal and middle thirds of the clavicle toward the contralateral nipple
   D. At the apex of the junction of the two heads of the sternocleidomastoid toward the ipsilateral nipple
   E. Under the posterior belly of the sternocleidomastoid muscle 1 cm above the clavicle toward the sternal notch

2. The tip of the catheter is in the:
   A. Mediastinum
   B. Right ventricle
   C. Right atrium
   D. Superior vena cava
   E. Brachiocephalic vein

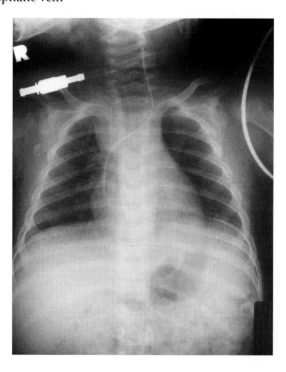

DISCUSSION

ANSWERS:

1. D. At the apex of the junction of the two heads of the sternocleidomastoid toward the ipsilateral nipple.
2. C. Right atrium

1. The catheter was placed in the internal jugular vein by inserting the needle at the apex of the triangle formed by the sternal and clavicular heads of the sternocleidomastoid muscle and aiming towards the ipsilateral nipple.

2. The tip of the catheter lies in the right atrium. It is obviously within the vascular system, as it courses from the internal jugular vein through the brachiocephalic vein and superior vena cava into the right atrium.

Further Discussion

Several approaches provide access to the internal jugular vein. One technique, used in this child, is described above. Anatomically, the internal jugular vein lies anterior and lateral to the carotid artery within the triangle formed by the two heads of the sternocleidomastoid muscle. Aiming toward the ipsilateral nipple serves to direct the needle away from the artery. The position of the catheter tip in the right atrium is acceptable, although some prefer placement in the superior vena cava or at the junction of the superior vena cava with the right atrium.

This 8-year-old boy has had a rash for 10 days. He has been taking a medicine each morning for the last 3 weeks due to a swollen scalp area where his hair fell out.

1. The most likely medicine is:
   A. Cephalexin
   B. Prednisone
   C. Erythromycin
   D. Griseofulvin
   E. Fluconazole

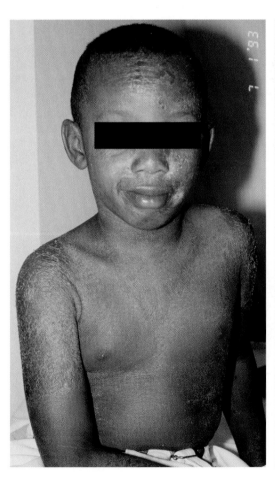
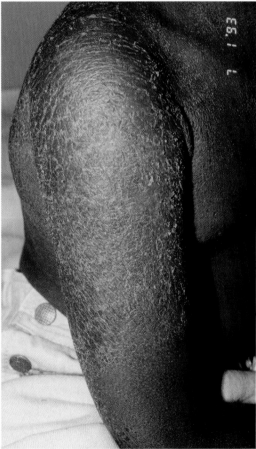

DISCUSSION

ANSWER:

1. **D. Griseofulvin**

1. His swollen scalp area with localized alopecia is likely to be due to tinea capitis and kerion formation. Cephalexin might be used to treat a bacterial cellulitis but is not effective for fungal infections and is taken 2 to 4 times a day. An allergic reaction to cephalexin usually causes an urticarial rash which this child does not have. Prednisone is occasionally used to treat kerions, but only along with an antifungal agent. Erythromycin is not used for fungal infections and its administration is only very rarely associated with allergic reactions. Fluconazole is generally reserved for more severe fungal infections than tinea capitis or for patients in whom conventional antifungal therapy is unsuccessful. In addition, the safety and efficacy of fluconazole in patients less than 13 years of age has not been established. The correct answer is griseofulvin.

Further Discussion

Topical antifungal agents are usually ineffective against tinea capitis since they do not penetrate to the hair bulb. Oral griseofulvin is an antifungal agent that is deposited in keratin precursor cells. The new fungal-free cells replace the infected hair, making this drug effective for tinea capitis. It can be administered once a day for 4 to 8 weeks but is associated with hypersensitivity rashes. These rashes may consist of typical urticaria, angioedema, toxic epidermal necrolysis, photosensitivity, or generalized desquamation, as in this patient.

The mother of a 3-week-old girl reports that her child developed drainage from her umbilicus since the remnant of her cord separated 1 week ago. The infant has been otherwise well. Specifically, she has not had fever, vomiting, or diarrhea. On examination, she is vigorous and afebrile.

1. When you swab this area, you get secretions that are:
   A. Feculent
   B. Bloody
   C. Serous
   D. Purulent
   E. Uriniferous

2. Culture of this lesion might yield:
   A. *Escherichia coli*
   B. *Staphylococcus aureus*
   C. *Staphylococcus epidermidis*
   D. None of the above
   E. All of the above

3. Treatment for this lesion relies on:
   A. Intravenous antibiotics
   B. Incision and drainage
   C. Topical antibiotics
   D. Silver nitrate
   E. Surgical correction

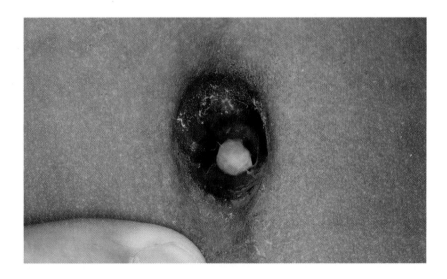

DISCUSSION

ANSWERS:

1. C. Serous
2. E. All of the above
3. D. Silver nitrate

1. This baby has an umbilical granuloma, which may form when the cord separates at 10-14 days of age and leads to serous discharge. Other disorders in this anatomic region include omphalitis, a patent urachus (connecting to the bladder), and a patent omphalomesenteric duct (connecting to the bowel). Omphalitis is characterized by circumferential erythema, induration around the umbilicus, and a purulent discharge, generally in an acutely ill infant. Both a urachus and an omphalomesenteric duct may have an obvious tract and a distinctive discharge.

2. Since an umbilical granuloma is not infectious in nature, your swab will yield normal flora for a newborn that includes staphylococcal and coliform species. Omphalitis is most often caused by *S. aureus* and less often by gram-negative enteric rods.

3. Judicious application of silver nitrate treats an umbilical granuloma. For omphalitis, intravenous antibiotics are indicated; oxacillin and gentamicin would provide appropriate coverage. A patent urachus or omphalomesenteric duct is repaired surgically.

Further Discussion

Umbilical granulomas occur frequently. They are characterized by a scant serous discharge and are contained within the area of the umbilicus. In all cases, one must be certain that the problem is not omphalitis, which causes a purulent discharge and the appearance of erythema and induration in the peri-umbilical area.

An 18-month-old boy, visiting the United States from Ireland, is brought to the emergency department by his aunt. He is previously healthy except for a seizure disorder for which he takes phenytoin. His aunt states that he awoke with a "rash" and denies any systemic illness or recent trauma.

1. Your diagnosis is
    A. Staphylococcal scalded skin syndrome
    B. Scald burn
    C. Erythema multiforme
    D. Drug eruption
    E. None of the above

2. Treatment includes:
    A. Intravenous saline
    B. Topical Silvadene
    C. Intravenous prednisone
    D. Intravenous oxacillin
    E. Oral prednisolone

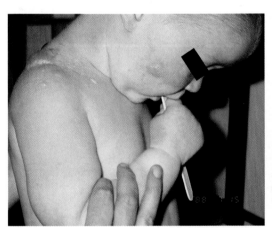
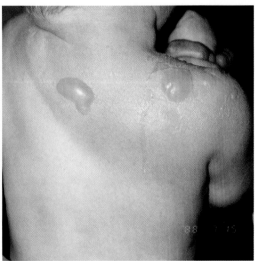

DISCUSSION

ANSWERS:

1. E. None of the above
2. B. Topical Silvadene

1. This fair-haired young lad came to America from his home in Ireland on July 14 and promptly joined his cousins in the pool the next afternoon (as indicated at the bottom of the illustration). When his tee shirt got wet, it slid down over one shoulder, and he developed a second degree sunburn. While a scald burn shares some features with a sunburn, several findings rule against hot water as the source of the injury. If the mechanism were a splash, one would expect less confluence and the typical pattern of satellite lesions. On the other hand, it is difficult to imagine that an immersion involving the neck and shoulders would spare most of the face and head. The characteristic target lesions of erythema multiforme are not present, and a drug reaction is not likely to lead to a localized bullous eruption. Thus, none of the answers is correct. You may wish to give yourself partial credit for selecting "Scald Burns," but I would not be so generous in this case.

2. Many regimens are acceptable for the management of small burns on an ambulatory basis, and Silvadene is certainly among them. For a second degree burn that involves perhaps 5% of the body surface area, admission and intravenous fluids are not appropriate. Oxacillin might play a role in staphylococcal scalded skin syndrome, and steroids are used in selected cases of erythema multiforme and drug eruption.

A 16-year-old with severe acne complains that his tongue "looks funny."

1. What may predispose the patient to this disorder?
    A. Corticosteroid therapy
    B. A steady diet of junk food
    C. Antimicrobial treatment
    D. Pustular psoriasis
    E. Immunodeficiency

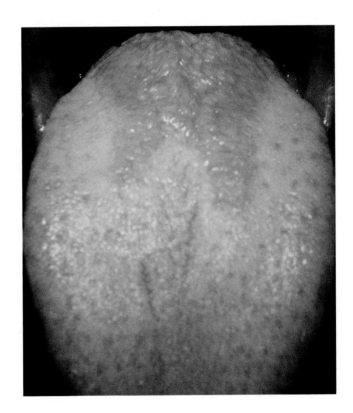

DISCUSSION

ANSWER:

1. C. Antimicrobial treatment

1. Corticosteroids, systemic or inhaled, or immunodeficiency may predispose a patient to oral candidiasis, which is usually manifested by white patches on the buccal mucosa. A steady diet of junk food may not be ideal, but should not really affect his tongue. Pustular psoriasis can be associated with tongue involvement, but patients with this condition usually have a history of psoriasis, a high fever and signs of acute illness, and irregular lines of ulceration and atrophy of the filiform papillae of the tongue, not the "hairy" appearance seen here. This patient has black hairy tongue, or in this case, a sort of brown hairy tongue. This condition is associated with systemic antimicrobials, such as tetracycline, which may be prescribed for acne vulgaris.

Further Discussion

Black hairy tongue is a disorder of unclear etiology characterized by a dark matted coating on the posterior aspect of the tongue. The filiform papillae are elongated, often in a triangular area just anterior to the circumvallate papillae. It is associated with poor oral hygiene, smoking, and systemic antimicrobials. Initial therapy should consist of stopping any predisposing activities or agents, and gently brushing the tongue with a soft toothbrush.

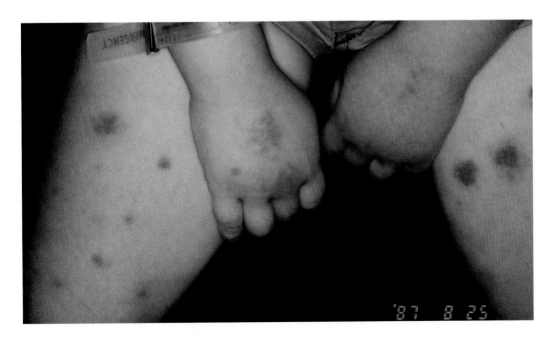

CASE 63

A 5-year-old boy has been sick for 5 days. His illness began with a fever that resolved on the third day. The day prior to this visit, a rash developed. Today he complained of difficulty walking.

Vital signs	P 98/min R 18/min BP 105/55 mm Hg T 37.8°C
General	No distress
HEENT	Clear
Nodes	Shoddy cervical adenopathy
Lungs	No rales
Heart	Sinus tachycardia, no murmurs or rubs
Abdomen	Nontender, no hepatomegaly or splenomegaly

1. A complete blood count shows:
   A. 25,000/mm^3 platelets
   B. 10% lymphoblasts
   C. 1% reticulocytes
   D. 15% atypical lymphocytes
   E. 25% hematocrit

2. The boy develops a complication the following day that requires treatment with:
   A. An enema
   B. Gamma globulin
   C. Antibiotics
   D. Dialysis
   E. Transfusion

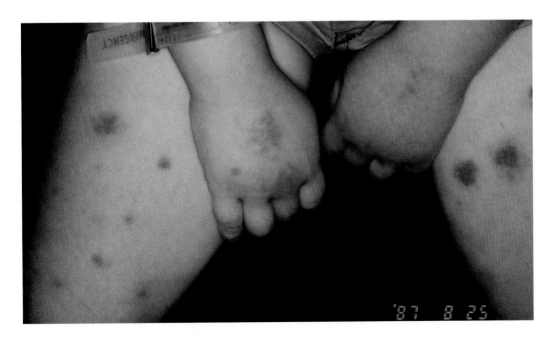

DISCUSSION

ANSWERS:

1. C. 1% reticulocytes
2. A. An enema

1. The photograph shows a well-perfused 5-year-old boy with purpuric lesions, including on the lower extremities, and edema of the dorsum of his hands. Given the history, one might consider Henoch Schönlein purpura (HSP), which he has, as well as idiopathic thrombocytopenic purpura, hemolytic uremic syndrome (HUS), and leukemia. None of these entities, except HSP, should cause both the purpura and the edema. The lack of a history of bloody diarrhea and anuria weighs against HUS. With leukemia, the fever would likely have persisted and one might find lymph node enlargement and/or hepatosplenomegaly.

   Given that this is HSP, a vasculitis rather than a disease of the blood, the CBC should be completely normal. Of the values given, only the reticulocytes fall in the normal range.

2. When the child with HSP develops abdominal pain, vasculitis is the usual cause but one must consider intussusception. This well known complication is both diagnosed and treated (in 50-75% of cases) with a contrast enema, using either air or barium.

Further Discussion

Although some physicians may think that HSP is always limited to the buttocks and lower extremities, as illustrated here this is not the case. Purpura and arthritis may occur more diffusely. Once the differential diagnosis has been narrowed down to HSP, the key to management is the presence or absence of significant renal disease. Children with normal renal function and no hypertension can be managed as outpatients. They should be followed closely for monitoring of blood pressure and urinary sediment and instructed to return if severe or persistent abdominal pain develops. Since HSP may linger for weeks, it is advisable to share the expected duration with the family.

A 3-year-old uncircumcised boy is brought to your attention because of pain and swelling of his penis. He has been well except for a slight upper respiratory infection. His mother denies any recent trauma but reports that he spent the weekend with his father. The child was well several hours ago. There is no history of frequency, dysuria, or hematuria.

1. Your diagnosis is:
    A. Priapism
    B. Phimosis
    C. Balanoposthitis
    D. Nephrotic syndrome
    E. Paraphimosis

2. Based on this you would:
    A. Refer to a urologist
    B. Treat with antibiotics
    C. Manually reduce
    D. Check a urinalysis
    E. Report as suspected sexual abuse

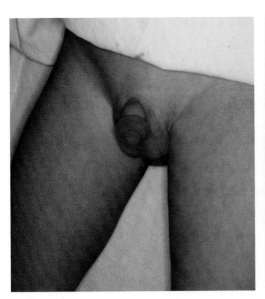
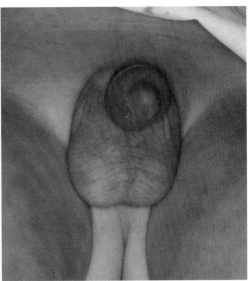

DISCUSSION

ANSWERS:

1. E. Paraphimosis
2. C. Manually reduce

1. The findings are consistent with the diagnosis of paraphimosis, which occurs when the foreskin is retracted over the glans. As edema and venous congestion ensue, the return of the foreskin to its natural position is inhibited. Phimosis is a condition that exists when tightness of the distal foreskin precludes its being withdrawn to expose the glans. Balanoposthitis is an infection of the foreskin that may extend onto the glans. It is a form of cellulitis that begins with a break or crack in the skin. In both these conditions, the foreskin, which will be in the normal position, covers the glans. Priapism is prolonged painful erection unaccompanied by sexual stimulation. The major underlying causes are trauma, leukemic infiltrate or sickle cell disease. While nephrotic syndrome may produce swelling in the genital area, it involves the scrotum, rather than the penis, as an extension of ascites.

2. By applying pressure over the glans and steady traction on the foreskin, a paraphimosis can be easily reduced in the vast majority of cases. Measures that may be of assistance include the application of ice to reduce the edema and the use of mineral oil and surgical lubricant. Sometimes a local anesthetic block or systemic sedation facilitates the procedure. Only rarely will urologic consultation be necessary to accomplish a surgical reduction. The existence of paraphimosis is not a specific alerting sign of child abuse. The foreskin is often retracted by the child. Thus to report this as suspected child abuse would be an error, unless there are some other indicators. While used for balanoposthitis, antibiotics have no role in this condition. A urinalysis, if performed, would be normal.

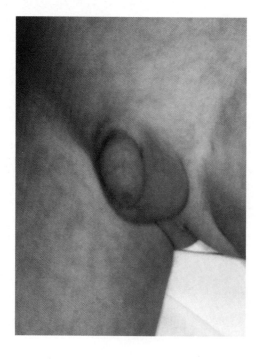

CASE 65

A father brings his 2-year-old son for "lumps" on his head. The lesions began 2 weeks earlier. Initially they were several millimeters in diameter, but some enlarged. New lesions have continued to appear. The father shaved the boy's hair over the affected area (causing a small amount of bleeding) to be able to wash the scalp more thoroughly, and brings him for evaluation, now that he is aware of the extent of the condition. The child has been in good health and has not had any fever or malaise. He has experienced no prior dermatologic problems. On examination, he is well appearing and afebrile. The anterior cervical nodes are mildly enlarged on his right side and nontender. He has no hepatosplenomegaly. Other than his scalp, the remainder of his skin is normal.

1. Your diagnosis is:
   A. Lymphoma
   B. Tinea capitis
   C. Folliculitis
   D. Seborrhea
   E. Job's syndrome

2. The test most likely to assist you is:
   A. IgE level
   B. Bone marrow biopsy
   C. Fungal culture
   D. IgG level
   E. Bacterial culture

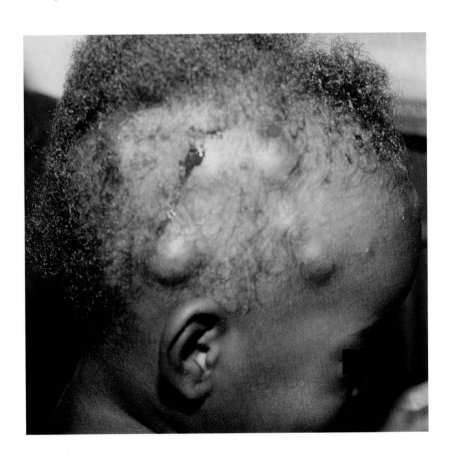

DISCUSSION

ANSWERS:

1. C. Folliculitis
2. E. Bacterial culture

1. This boy has folliculitis. Characteristic lesions, which are red papules with central pustular formation, are seen anteriorly just above the forehead. More posteriorly, the lesions have evolved into furuncles. Tinea capitis takes several forms: alopecia, broken hairs ("black dot" tinea), dandruff, and kerion formation. The only variety producing an appearance similar to the scalp of this child would be multiple kerions, which are usually exudative and covered with matted hair and debris. Seborrhea causes a greasy, scaly scalp, but not discrete follicular lesions and furuncles. In cases of Job's syndrome, furuncles occur frequently in all regions of the body and recur, rather than affecting just one site at a given point in time. Lymphoma in childhood does not cause localized lesions, such as these; additionally, the individual furuncles here appear tense and fluctuant, rather than firm and neoplastic.

2. Treatment for the larger furuncles requires incision and drainage in addition to local measures and systemic antibiotics. While *Staphylococcus aureus* is far and away the most likely isolate, culture of the material obtained at the time of drainage makes sense to confirm the etiology and guide the selection of antibiotics. On the other hand, I would not usually culture a single furuncle in an otherwise healthy patient. Fungal culture is helpful to diagnose suspected tinea, when the appearance is atypical, bone marrow biopsy is indicated in patients with hematogenous malignancies, and IgE levels are abnormally elevated with Job's syndrome. In certain immunodeficiencies other than Job's syndrome, IgG levels are low.

Further Discussion

This is an usually severe case of folliculitis. In general, one encounters only scattered pustular lesions. However, some cases become more pronounced, as seen here, usually in the absence of any specific underlying condition.

A 12-year-old comes to the emergency department with a history of intermittent palpitations. Earlier that day he reported that he felt his heart pounding rapidly and experienced chest tightness and dizziness.

1. What caused his palpitations?
   A. Ventricular tachycardia
   B. Hypoglycemia
   C. Supraventricular tachycardia
   D. Atrial flutter
   E. Hyperthyroidism

2. Initial therapy for his underlying disorder might include:
   A. Adenosine.
   B. Cardioversion
   C. Digoxin
   D. Propranolol
   E. Propylthiouracil

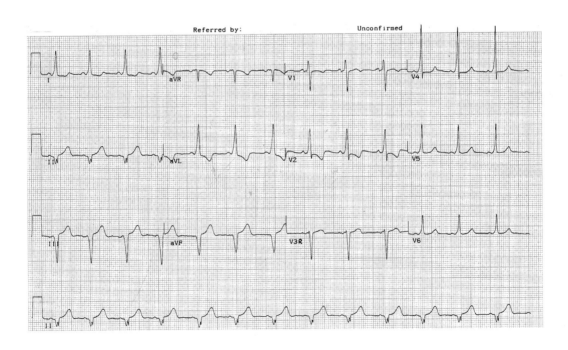

DISCUSSION

ANSWERS:

1. **C. Supraventricular tachycardia**
2. **D. Propranolol**

1. The tracing shows sinus rhythm and Wolff-Parkinson-White syndrome (WPW) with short PR intervals, a wide QRS complex and delta waves. There is left axis deviation, secondary to WPW. Although a short, spontaneously remitting run of ventricular tachycardia may have caused the patient's symptoms, ventricular tachycardia is not associated with the WPW pre-excitation syndromes. Patients with hypoglycemia may present with near syncope but the palpitations, lack of diaphoresis, mental status changes, and current EKG make this unlikely. Atrial flutter does not usually spontaneously remit and, in older children, is usually associated with congenital heart disease resulting in stretched atria such as mitral or tricuspid insufficiency or intra-atrial surgery. The spontaneous resolution of the tachycardia and the lack of exophthalmos, goiter, tremor, or hypertension make hyperthyroidism unlikely. The patient's spontaneously resolving tachycardia could have been a supraventricular tachycardia (SVT), ectopic atrial tachycardia, atrial flutter, atrial fibrillation or a ventricular tachycardia. The spontaneous resolution and the current EKG suggest SVT, caused by his WPW syndrome.

2. Adenosine and cardioversion are used to manage acute SVT but are not indicated when the SVT has resolved. Patients with SVT due to WPW should not receive digoxin because it may increase the rate of bypass tract conduction. Propylthiouracil may be used to treat hyperthyroidism. Patients with SVT and WPW are usually controlled with a single drug such as propranolol, procainamide, or flecainide.

Further Discussion

WPW is the most common of the pre-excitation syndromes and results from conduction through an anomalous path (the Kent bundle) between the atrium and the ventricle. The part of the ventricle attached to the anomalous pathway is depolarized prematurely and slowly producing the short PR and the slurred upstroke of the QRS (the delta wave). A premature systole transmitted through the A-V node is conducted in a retrograde manner back up the anomalous tract to the atrium. This action can initiate the tachycardia since the bypass tract has a shorter refractory period than the A-V node.

This 7-year-old girl complains of sore throat and fever for 3 days. She denies headache, conjunctivitis, rhinorrhea, or cough. On examination, her temperature is 39°C. She has bilaterally enlarged, mildly tender anterior cervical lymph nodes. Her lungs are clear to auscultation and percussion. No cardiac murmurs are heard. You do not appreciate abdominal tenderness or organomegaly.

1. Which of the following statements is true?
   A. A "monospot" test has a 90% chance of being positive
   B. A viral throat culture has a 60% chance of being positive
   C. A bacterial throat culture has a 70% chance of being positive
   D. A streptococcal latex agglutination test has an 80% chance of being positive
   E. A test for IgM anti-VCA has a 95% chance of being positive

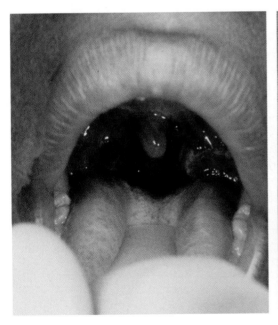 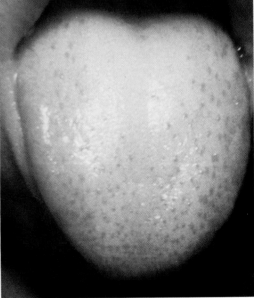

DISCUSSION

ANSWER:

1. **C. A bacterial throat culture has a 70% chance of being positive.**

1. The girl has streptococcal pharyngitis. Given her clinical findings, you can be about 80% certain of this diagnosis. Since culture is positive in 90% of patients with streptococcal pharyngitis, the correct answer here is about 70% (i.e., 90% of 80%). In culture proven cases of streptococcal pharyngitis, the latex agglutination test has a sensitivity of only 50-60%. Her illness has been brief in duration and she has no posterior cervical adenopathy or splenomegaly, making infectious mononucleosis unlikely. Even if she had mononucleosis, given that she is 7 years old and in the first week of her illness, a "monospot" test would only be positive 50-70% of the time under these conditions; the assay reaches a sensitivity of 90% for adolescents after 2 to 3 weeks of illness. IgM anti-VCA, while highly specific for Epstein Barr virus, even early in the course of disease, is not nearly as sensitive as the "monospot" test for typical cases. Viral pharyngitis is unlikely with this clinical picture. In cases of pharyngitis where tests for other pathogens (e.g., Group A streptococci, Epstein Barr virus) are negative, only 15-20% will have a positive viral culture.

Further Discussion

Group A beta hemolytic streptococci cause 30-50% of pharyngitis in school-age children, and are occasional pathogens in younger patients, but generally not before 2 years of age. The classic findings in this infection include high fever, beefy red tonsils with a whitish exudate, palatal petechiae, tender anterior cervical nodes, and the absence of the usual findings in a viral upper respiratory infection, specifically conjunctivitis and rhinorrhea. My approach is to treat, without testing, the small percentage of school-age children with an absolutely typical constellation of signs and symptoms, since clinical diagnosis is 80-85% accurate. In these circumstances, culture only adds 5-10% more, and it has a 10% false-negative rate. For patients over 2 years old with any degree of inflammation in the posterior pharynx, I perform a rapid latex agglutination assay and prescribe antibiotics when the result is positive. If this test is negative, I recommend symptomatic measures and await the report on the culture. Because children in the first 2 years of life are highly unlikely to have streptococcal pharyngitis, and have been described only rarely to develop nonsuppurative complications, I do not conduct studies in those with only mild erythema but follow the approach above when I see exudate or palatal petechiae.

This 2-year-old has had 4 days of fever and lesions progressing from the mouth and tongue to the perioral skin up to the right eyelid. The child had chickenpox at 1 year of age. She is afebrile and generally well appearing. The remainder of her skin is clear.

1. The agent most likely to cause these lesions is:
   A. Group A *Streptococcus*
   B. Varicella zoster virus
   C. Coxsackie A16 virus
   D. Herpes simplex type 1
   E. *Staphylococcus aureus*

2. A potential complication from this problem is:
   A. Chronic facial pain
   B. Glomerulonephritis
   C. Myocarditis
   D. Corneal ulceration
   E. Mitral regurgitation

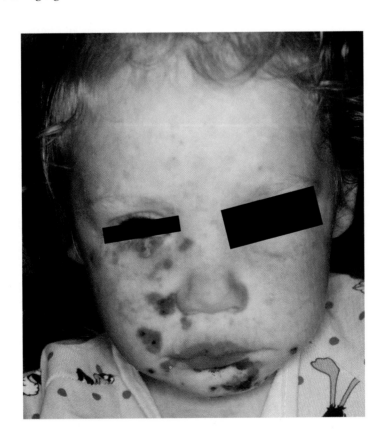

DISCUSSION

ANSWERS:
1. **D. Herpes simplex type 1**
2. **D. Corneal ulceration**

1. This child has herpes simplex type 1, initially involving the mouth with autoinoculation of the face. Group A streptococcal and staphylococcal impetigo can cause facial infections with yellow crusts like some of these lesions. However, impetigo does not involve the oral cavity, but more likely originates at the nares. The varicella zoster virus can cause a recurrent infection (shingles) in normal children. The rash consists of painful vesicles and papules on an erythematous base extending along the dermatome of the infected nerve root or cranial nerve ganglia. This is unlikely to be shingles because the rash does not extend in a band and it involves more than one division of the trigeminal (fifth) nerve. The oral cavity and skin below the mouth are innervated by the mandibular nerve, V-3, and this child has lesions on both sides of the midline below the mouth. The maxillary nerve (V-2) innervates the skin between the mouth and lower eyelid. Involvement of the ophthalmic branch (V-1) could damage the cornea, but this only occurs when the nasociliary branch is involved and is manifested by vesicles on the skin over the nose. Coxsackie virus may cause vesicles and ulcers of the posterior pharynx as well as the hands and feet, but not the face as in this child. Herpes simplex is a common viral infection during childhood, with type 1 predominately causing oral infections and type 2 usually genital infections. The lesions begin as vesicles, initially in most cases involving the tongue, gingiva, and lips. As the disease progresses, the lesions progress to erythematous ulcerations and hemorrhage and may spread to the perioral skin. Fever and cervical lymphadenopathy are common.

2. A potential complication of this child's infection is corneal ulceration. Impetigo may be complicated by glomerulonephritis, but only streptococcal pharyngitis can lead to rheumatic fever, manifest by mitral or aortic valve damage. Coxsackie viruses are one of the more common agents recovered from patients with myocarditis. Although chronic facial pain may follow herpes zoster of the fifth cranial nerve, it is rarely seen in children.

Further Discussion

Herpes simplex may infect the eye, potentially causing annoying recurrences and/or compromising vision. One should consider this agent in any child with conjunctivitis, particularly when the infection is unilateral or accompanied by cutaneous vesicles. To make the diagnosis, fluorescein is instilled into the eye to look for the characteristic dendritic ulcerations. Treatment for corneal involvement requires topical antiviral therapy and close follow up.

This child fell 5 feet from a tree branch to the ground the evening before seeking medical attention. He arrived at 10:00 PM with his arm in a sling, complaining of pain throughout the upper extremity. On examination, his elbow was mildly swollen and tender. His radial pulse and distal sensation were intact.

1. The 5 arrows point to:
   A. Subcutaneous emphysema
   B. A hematoma
   C. A fat pad
   D. Joint fluid
   E. A fascial plane

2. Your diagnosis is:
   A. Radial head dislocation
   B. Radial head fracture
   C. Sprained elbow
   D. Nursemaid's elbow
   E. Supracondylar fracture

3. Appropriate treatment for this injury in the emergency department is a:
   A. Short arm cast
   B. Posterior splint
   C. Shoulder immobilizer
   D. Sling and swathe
   E. Figure-of-eight bandage

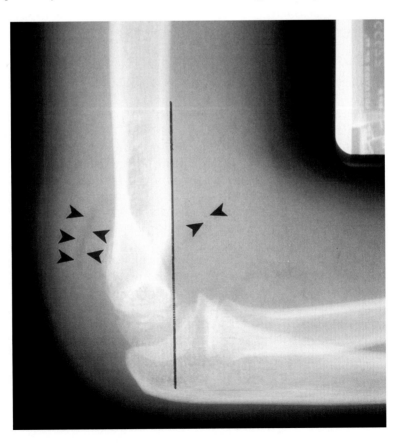

DISCUSSION

ANSWERS:
1. **C. A fat pad**
2. **E. Supracondylar fracture**
3. **B. Posterior splint**

1. The cluster of 5 arrows point to a posterior fat pad and the 2 other arrows point to a less well-visualized anterior fat pad. A posterior fat pad indicates the presence of a fracture, manifesting with blood in the joint space, and is never normal. An anterior fat pad may be visualized adjacent to the humerus when no injury is present, but if it is moved away from the bone it also indicates a fracture. The anterior humeral line should intersect the middle of the capitellum and is useful in assessing the degree of displacement of a supracondylar fracture.

2. This child has a supracondylar fracture, based on the presence and position of the fat pads, even though it is difficult to visualize a bony defect. The radial head is not dislocated, as it points toward the capitellum, and no fracture of the radius is seen. Nursemaid's elbow (subluxed radial head) does not cause the visualization of a posterior fat pad. One should be leery of diagnosing a sprain of the elbow in a child with open physes, and this injury would also not lead to the appearance of a posterior fat pad.

3. The appropriate emergency treatment is a posterior splint and prompt communication with an orthopedist, due to concern about Volkmann's ischemic contracture. While a long arm cast provides definitive treatment, a short arm cast would serve no purpose whatsoever. A figure-of-eight bandage is a treatment for fracture of the clavicle. Neither a shoulder immobilizer nor a sling and swathe adequately immobilize this injury.

Further Discussion

Supracondylar fractures account for over 50% of the fractures of the elbow in pediatrics, usually affecting children between 3 and 10 years of age. Complications occur frequently and include immediate neurovascular compromise and long term deformities. The main priorities for the emergency physician are neurovascular assessment and immobilization. Vascular assessment begins with palpation of the distal pulses and measurement of capillary refill, and proceeds to the use of a Doppler ultrasound device to detect flow, if necessary. One needs to keep in mind, however, that significant muscle ischemia can occur even when the pulses and capillary refill appear to be adequate. Function of the radial, ulnar, and median nerves should be tested. Prompt placement of a posterior splint helps to limit ongoing tissue injury and edema formation, which is very important since this area is susceptible to vascular injury.

There are several schema for classifying supracondylar fractures. I prefer to use the categories described in the table, as they are descriptive, easy to remember, and convey information with implications for choice of therapy.

TYPE	APPEARANCE	DIAGNOSIS
I	Nondisplaced	Fat pad sign, fracture line not visible
II	Displaced, with intact posterior cortex	Fracture line, ant. humeral line abnormal
III	Displaced, with no cortical contact	Obvious fracture with displacement

A 12-year-old girl complains of intermittent severe headaches for 3 days. She has experienced no fever, neck pain, weakness, or incoordination.

Vital signs:	P 82/min R 18/min BP 190/130 mm Hg T 37.1°C
General	No distress
HEENT	No facial tenderness. PERRLA, EOMI, disks flat. No rhinorrhea. Dentition noncarious.
Nodes	Shoddy cervical adenopathy
Lungs	No rales or wheezes
Heart	Sinus tachycardia, no murmurs or rubs
Abdomen	Nontender, no hepatomegaly or splenomegaly
Neurologic	Alert, oriented x 3. No focal findings

Hgb 12.3 gm/dl, Hct 37%, WBC 10,800/mm³, Platelets 228,000/mm³
S.G. 1.018, pH 5.2, RBC 50-100/ hpf, WBC 0-1/hpf, Bacteria negative

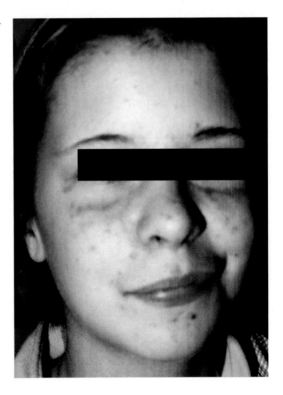

1. Thumbing through the patient's prior laboratory data on the computer you find:
   A. Positive LE prep and high complement
   B. Positive ASO titer and positive ANA
   C. Positive ANA and low complement
   D. Positive LE prep and negative ANA
   E. Positive rheumatoid factor and elevated ASO titer

2. You decide to treat this patient as follows:
   A. Referral to a nephrologist
   B. Sublingual nifedipine
   C. Oral hydralazine
   D. Intravenous furosemide
   E. Oral propanolol

DISCUSSION

ANSWERS:
1. C. Positive ANA and low complement
2. B. Sublingual nifedipine

1. This preteenage girl has the malar "butterfly" rash characteristic of lupus erythematosus, along with renal involvement. Over 90% of patients with lupus have a positive ANA and a large proportion have a positive LE prep. Elevated ASO titers follow infections with Group A streptococci and occur with post-streptococcal glomerulonephritis. Rheumatoid factor appears in certain forms of juvenile rheumatoid arthritis and occasionally in patients with systemic lupus erythematosus. Both post-streptococcal and lupus nephritis lead to the consumption of complement. Fitting all these elements together, the record is likely to show a positive ANA and hypocomplementemia in this patient with lupus nephritis.

2. With a diastolic pressure of 130 mm Hg in a patient with headaches and lupus nephritis, you have a hypertensive emergency on your hands. Referral is unnecessary and any delay could prove fatal. Neither oral hydralazine nor oral propanolol will act sufficiently fast. Similarly, intravenous diuretic administration is not an acceptable choice. I would start with 10 mg of sublingual nifedipine or treat intravenously with nitroprusside, diazoxide, or labetolol. Although controversy about sublingual nifedipine has been raised, I am comfortable using it in this situation and have found the drug to be effective without any adverse effects. Intravenous hydralazine, although marginally slower in onset, would be a reasonable option if you are certain the patient has no changes consistent with hypertensive injury on fundoscopic examination, as this would mandate a more potent drug.

Further Discussion

Although lupus erythematosus and other collagen vascular diseases are chronic illnesses that are managed primarily by physicians in their offices, emergent complications occur on occasion. Particularly important considerations include infections, seizures, pericarditis, pleural effusion, peritonitis, nephritis, hypertension, and hemolytic anemia.

CASE 71

The mother of a 1-year-old brings him to the emergency department with the acute onset of respiratory distress. The child ate dinner at 6 PM and immediately thereafter felt warm. His temperature was 39.5°C. Over the next 2 hours his breathing became increasing "noisy" and his fever persisted. He is in your emergency department now at 10 PM Past medical history is remarkable for the fact that the child has not been immunized due to his family's religious beliefs. His vitals signs are: P 150/min, R 36/min, BP 95/50 mm Hg, and T 40.1°C. You hear stridor while he is at rest. He refuses to open his mouth, so you delay examination of the oropharynx. There is minimal anterior cervical adenopathy and the lungs are clear.

1. Which of the following is the least likely diagnosis?
   A. Croup
   B. Epiglottitis
   C. Diphtheria
   D. Retropharyngeal abscess
   E. Peritonsillar abscess

2. Which of the following is the most likely diagnosis?
   A. Croup
   B. Epiglottitis
   C. Diphtheria
   D. Retropharyngeal abscess
   E. Peritonsillar abscess

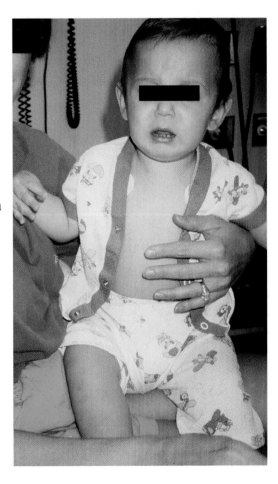

3. The child becomes agitated when you start your examination. How would you manage him?
   A. Administer racemic epinephrine and observe for 3 hours
   B. Send him to radiology for a soft tissue lateral neck X-ray
   C. Consult otolaryngology for an emergent intubation in the OR
   D. Hold him down and examine his throat with a tongue depressor
   E. None of the above

While waiting to obtain a portable lateral neck X-ray, the child develops increasing respiratory distress and becomes cyanotic. You attempt to manually ventilate him unsuccessfully and proceed with laryngoscopy and intubation. At laryngoscopy, you make the diagnosis.

4. Your diagnosis is:
    A. Epiglottitis
    B. Retropharyngeal abscess
    C. Croup
    D. Peritonsillar abscess
    E. Aspirated foreign body

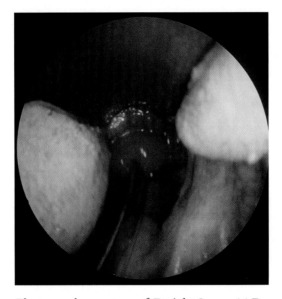

Photograph courtesy of Dwight Jones, M.D., Department of Otolaryngology, Children's Hospital, Boston, Massachusetts.

DISCUSSION

ANSWERS:

1. E. Peritonsillar abscess
2. B. Epiglottitis
3. E. None of the above
4. A. Epiglottitis

1. Croup, epiglottitis, retropharyngeal abscess, and diphtheria cause fever and stridor. Patients with peritonsillar infections are febrile but usually have a muffled, or "hot potato," voice rather than stridor. Both peritonsillar abscess and epiglottitis occur more frequently in older children; this is particularly true for peritonsillar abscess. Although epidemic in Russia at the time of this writing, diphtheria occurs rarely in the Untied States, even among patients who have not been immunized. Additionally, the onset is more gradual in most cases than described here, and massive enlargement of the cervical lymph nodes usually occurs. Given the clinical finding of stridor and the age of this patient, peritonsillar abscess becomes the least likely diagnosis, but diphtheria is the rarest epidemiologically. Since this is not a test scored by a computer, but rather a learning exercise, either answer is acceptable.

2. Once again, the same entities listed above cause fever and stridor. The age of the child points to croup or a retropharyngeal infection. On the other hand, the abrupt onset favors epiglottitis, with retropharyngeal abscess in second place. The child is not extremely toxic in appearance, most compatible with croup, yet he proceeds to obstruct before your eyes, which suggests epiglottitis. I'll concede that some conflicting clues are present, which is what happens when one describes real patients; nevertheless, I'll cast my vote strongly for epiglottitis, based on the rapid onset, high fever, and sudden respiratory arrest. Some children have a less toxic clinical appearance than suggested by the textbooks, and a proportion of the cases occur, as described in the pre-Hib vaccine era, in patients both younger and older than the classic 3 to 7-year-old range. Take half-credit for either croup or retropharyngeal abscess. After all, this is a book of pictures and this picture does not look like epiglottitis, despite the fact that the child had this disease.

3. The best choice is none of the above. Epiglottitis must cross your mind in this unimmunized child with the rapid onset of high fever and stridor, so please refrain from shoving a tongue depressor down his throat. Similarly, don't allow him to disappear into the abyss of radiology with only his mother and a technologist in attendance. Croup seems sufficiently unlikely to make the administration of racemic epinephrine a less than optimal choice, particularly without visualizing his posterior pharynx, which we just decided was a risky maneuver in this case (but not in the typical infant with croup). You could send him off to the operating room with an otolaryngologist, but this seems a bit extreme in a 1-year-old sitting on his mother's lap. Croup is hundreds of times more common than epiglottitis, even in unimmunized children, and some cases of croup cause the temperature to rise above 40°C. Thus, the correct approach is to either obtain a portable, soft tissue lateral neck in the emergency department or to have a physician skilled in airway management accompany the child to radiology.

4. This is the classic swollen, "cherry red" epiglottis seen in epiglottitis. In all the other conditions on this list, the supraglottic structures (epiglottis, ary-epiglottic folds, and arytenoids) are normal. Croup causes edema and inflammation of the vocal cords; retropharyngeal abscess produces a purulent mass in the posterior pharynx and peritonsillar abscess fills one of the tonsillar beds with pus. No foreign body is seen here.

CASE 72

A 5-year-old was playing with his sibling, who unintentionally discharged a pellet gun while he was standing just 5 feet away. The parents were immediately aware of the situation and contacted the emergency department for advice. They were told to call the local EMS service and have the child brought in for evaluation. On arrival, the child is awake and alert. The primary survey is normal and his vital signs are as follows: P 80/min, R 20/min, BP 100/70 mm Hg, and T 37°C. On secondary survey, the entire exam is normal except for the finding on his right side as shown below.

1. At this point you would:
    A. Probe the wound to see the extent of injury
    B. Repair the laceration and send the child home
    C. Observe the child for 6 hours
    D. Recommend surgical exploration
    E. Perform diagnostic peritoneal lavage

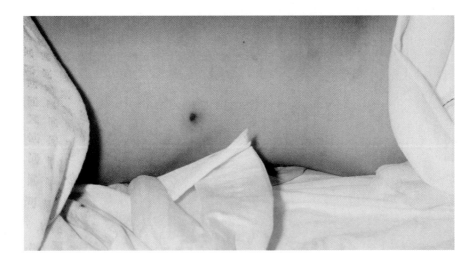

DISCUSSION

ANSWER:

1. D. Recommend surgical exploration

1. A reasonable choice is to recommend surgical exploration of the abdomen since a pellet gun discharged from close range is able to generate sufficient force to cause penetration of the peritoneum in most cases. One option, an abdominal CT scan, although not listed, is acceptable and was actually pursued prior to exploration, as this child had stable vital signs and was in a controlled setting. It showed a pellet embedded in the liver. Indications for diagnostic peritoneal lavage (DPL) are very rarely encountered. Only when a patient with multiple trauma requires an immediate neurosurgical procedure and there is also an immediate "need to know" about intra-abdominal bleeding is DPL performed. Probing the wound, observing the patient, or simply repairing the superficial laceration are all incorrect responses and pose a threat to the boy's safety, given the likelihood of penetration through the peritoneum and intra-abdominal injury. In addition to evaluating the abdominal wound, a chest X-ray is essential

Further Discussion

Progress in one domain does not always move us forward in others. Until recently pellet guns were relatively harmless, unless the projectile struck the eye. However, manufacturers recently developed "improved" models, capable of generating greater muzzle velocities. The new varieties of this "toy" are capable of propelling pellets through the abdominal wall, when fired from close range, such as within the confines of a room. Initially, a stable patient can be managed with imaging, supplemented by local exploration if the pellet appears to be located superficially on the images. If the pellet has penetrated the peritoneum or doubt exists, surgical consultation for potential exploration is warranted.

A 4-year-old previously healthy child has had a lump in the groin for 3 days. The swelling has increased in size. According to the mother, the child appears to be in pain. She denies fever, coughing, vomiting, diarrhea, or constipation. The family lives on a farm and keeps numerous pets. On examination, the temperature is 37.8°C; the positive findings are shown.

1. This problem is most likely caused by:
   A. A congenital defect
   B. *Staphylococcus aureus*
   C. Epstein Barr virus
   D. *Mycobacterium marinum*
   E. *Pasteurella multocida*

2. Appropriate treatment is:
   A. Oral isoniazid (INH) and rifampin
   B. Intravenous oxacillin
   C. Incision and drainage
   D. Oral prednisone
   E. Reduction in the OR

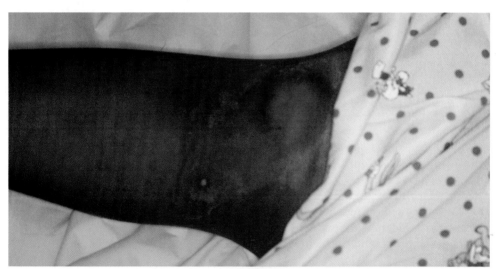

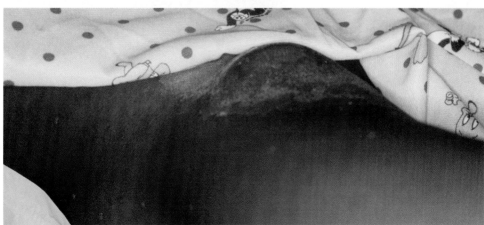

DISCUSSION

ANSWERS:
1. B. *Staphylococcus aureas*
2. C. **Incision and drainage**

1. This child has an infected inguinal lymph node, most likely caused by *S. aureus*. An isolated, enlarged lymph node is unlikely to be the result of a systemic infection due to Epstein Barr virus, the etiologic agent in infectious mononucleosis; additionally, the lymph nodes in this condition are covered by normal appearing skin. *M. marinum* causes "swimmer's granuloma," which is an unusual infection that generally arises on the distal extremities. Although *P. multocida* might be suspected based on the exposure to animals, this organism produces a wound infection rather than a lymphadenitis. Finally, an incarcerated inguinal hernia has a smooth, uninflamed surface. With progression to strangulation, the area might assume a more angry appearance, but one would expect the patient, at this point 3 days into the process, to be ill appearing and to have vomiting and abdominal distension.

2. The treatment for a fluctuant adenitis is incision and drainage. Although active against *S. aureus* and streptococci, intravenous oxacillin would not provide sufficient therapy for this localized collection of pus. INH and rifampin could be used to treat *M. marinum*, and prednisone is given to selected patients with infectious mononucleosis. Most hernias can be reduced in the emergency department and repaired electively at a later time in the operating room.

Further Discussion

A number of disease processes can cause swelling in the inguinal region. In addition to those mentioned above, sexually transmitted diseases figure prominently in the differential diagnosis in the adolescent. An unusual cause to consider with a rural exposure is plague due to *Yersinia pestis*.

One must be careful to exclude an incarcerated hernia before proceeding with incision and drainage or medical remedies for other conditions. Given the proximity of important neurovascular structures, drainage should be performed only by those familiar with the anatomy of the region and the technique.

CASE 74

A 4-year-old is brought to the emergency department for the problem of vigorous vomiting. The child has vomited many times and now has started to have diarrhea. The stool is profuse. The parent's have noted that the child has seemed weak, at times less responsive.

As you evaluate him you note: P 150/min, R 28/min, BP 80/40 mm Hg, T 38°C. He appears weak and somewhat unresponsive. His abdomen is distended. After starting an intravenous line and giving some rehydration fluids, you order the X-ray noted below.

1. Based on these findings you will look for which of the following immediate complications:
   A. Hypoglycemia
   B. Bowel stricture
   C. Metabolic alkalosis
   D. Seizures
   E. Hypertension

2. The next step in the management should be aimed at:
   A. Getting a stat blood level
   B. Decontamination
   C. Correcting prolonged coagulation studies
   D. Deferoxamine challenge test
   E. Activated charcoal

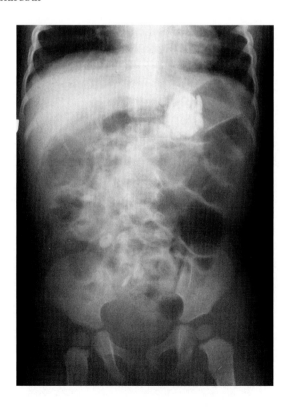

DISCUSSION

ANSWERS:

1. D. Seizures
2. B. Decontamination

1. The X-ray finding of opaque tablets matches the clinical manifestations (vomiting and hypotension), and the combination is diagnostic of iron poisoning. The consequences of this are bloody vomitus and diarrhea, shock, hyperglycemia, acidosis and central nervous system involvement, including coma and/or seizures. Bowel stricture, including pyloric stenosis, is a reported complication of iron poisoning, but it occurs late in the course (Phase IV), often several weeks after the ingestion.

2. The first step after fluid resuscitation is removal of the iron. This should be done by lavage with a large bore orogastric tube, and if there are residual tablets after gastric lavage, via bowel irrigation. Getting an iron level is important but it would not guide your initial management. The coagulation studies are also reasonable but do not supersede removal of the toxin, when this is the source if this problem. Deferoxamine challenge tests are helpful in asymptomatic patients. Other lab tests that may be suggestive of significant toxicity are serum glucose (elevated >150 mg/dl) and peripheral WBC count (>15,000/mm^3). Serial X-rays (figure below) may be helpful in examining the effectiveness of the decontamination and may also allow you to identify the number of pills ingested.

Further Discussion

Iron poisoning is still one of the most common life-threatening ingestions in children. Iron sulfate tablets look like candy and may be available in large numbers, particularly to children of women who are taking prenatal vitamins.

When the iron level report comes back, it is important to know that a finding of <350 micrograms/dl drawn 3 to 5 hours postingestion predicts an asymptomatic course. A level of 350-500 micrograms/dl will often be associated with symptoms, and a result of >500 micrograms/dl suggests significant risk for shock, coma, seizures and marked acidosis.

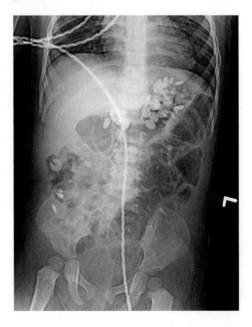

A 2-week-old is taken to the doctor because of concern about his umbilical cord. The cord has not fallen off and now it is emitting a strong odor. The infant is eating well but seems more cranky today. The parent's have not measured the temperature.

1. Based on these findings you would recommend:
   A. Topical antibiotic cream
   B. Alcohol wipes
   C. Oral cephalothin
   D. IV antibiotics
   E. Awaiting culture results

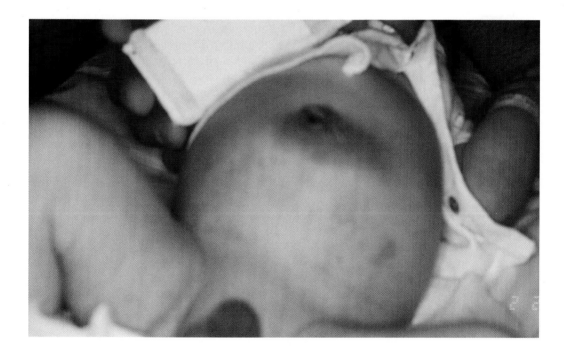

DISCUSSION

ANSWER:
1. **D. IV antibiotics**

1. This is a case of omphalitis, requiring admission to the hospital and treatment with IV antibiotics for both gram-positive and gram-negative organisms. When dealing with possible infections in newborns, a decision to await the results of cultures is often inappropriate. In that omphalitis is a form of cellulitis, neither cleansing with alcohol (sometimes recommended for infants who have minimal umbilical drainage without circumferential erythema and/or induration) nor the application of a topical antibiotic is sufficient.

Further Discussion

Omphalitis is characterized by purulent foul-smelling drainage from the cord and erythema that completely encircles the umbilicus. Because of the direct connection of the umbilicus to the central vascular system, systemic spread of the infection may occur rapidly. Thus, some infants may appear relatively well, while others may have a toxic appearance. All should be admitted and treated with oxacillin and gentamicin. The common organisms include *Streptococcus pyogenes, Staphylococcus aureus*, group B *Streptococcus*, and gram-negative enteric rods. Presentation in the first 2 weeks of life is characteristic. When there is any significance amount of drainage from the cord one must consider a vestigial attachment to the bladder or bowel, such as a patent urachus or omphalomesenteric duct.

The mother of a 3-year-old girl brings her to the emergency department for a rash, which began 24 hours earlier. She denies fever, lethargy, or malaise. The family lives in a suburb of Boston. The child has been healthy except for the recent diagnosis of a seizure disorder for which she is taking carbamazepine. On examination, she is afebrile with a pulse of 90/min and respirations of 18/min. She is in no distress and runs around the room during your examination. Other than a diffuse, patchy rash, most prominent on the ears, she has no abnormal physical findings.

1. Your diagnosis is:
    A. Meningococcemia
    B. Idiopathic thrombocytopenia
    C. Scarlet fever
    D. Drug reaction
    E. Henoch Schönlein purpura

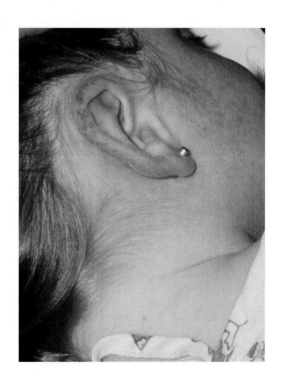

DISCUSSION

ANSWER:

1. **D. Drug reaction**

1. This is a drug eruption from carbamazepine (Tegretol®). While purpuric patches may be seen with meningococcemia, Rocky Mountain spotted fever (RMSF), or Henoch Schönlein purpura (HSP), the rest of the clinical picture does not fit. Patients with meningococcemia and RMSF are almost always febrile and most often ill-appearing. HSP affects predominantly the lower extremities and is often accompanied by edema and arthralgias or frank arthritis. This girl could conceivably have idiopathic thrombocytopenia (ITP), but one could not really make a diagnosis of ITP in a patient taking carbamazepine.

Further Discussion

The safest bet when a patient taking a drug develops a rash is to assume the rash has occurred as a reaction to the drug. This is very true for anticonvulsant medications in general and for carbamazepine in particular. Carbamazepine causes a number of cutaneous eruptions, from purpura to a life-threatening exfoliation. Purpura may occur secondary to either thrombocytopenia or vasculitis, with a normal platelet count. In this case, thrombocytopenia was not present. The lesions resolved following cessation of the carbamazepine.

A 14-year-old boy complains of pain in his leg for 3 days. He has felt fatigued, but denies fever or sore throat. His father thinks that he has been losing weight lately, but the boy attributes any changes to the fact that he's been engaged in a conditioning program with his football team. The picture shows his shin.

Vital signs:	P 72/min R 18/min BP 115/75 mm Hg T 37.1°C
General	No distress
HEENT	Pharynx without injection
Nodes	Shoddy cervical adenopathy
Lungs	No rales or wheezes
Heart	No murmurs or rubs
Abdomen	Mild tenderness in the periumbilical area; no rebound; active peristalsis
Neurologic	Alert, oriented x 3. No focal findings

1. The test most likely to yield an etiologic diagnosis is:
   A. Barium enema
   B. Cryptococcal antigen
   C. Chest X-ray
   D. Throat culture
   E. Biopsy of the lesion

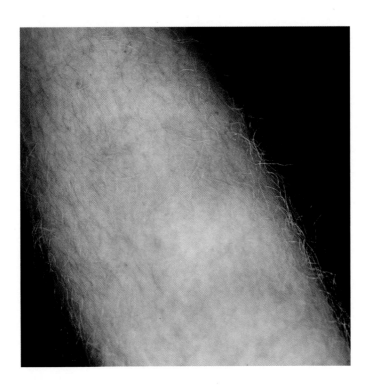

DISCUSSION

ANSWERS:

1. **A. Barium enema**

1. This boy has erythema nodosum. Given his age, a history of weight loss, and the finding of abdominal tenderness, inflammatory bowel disease is the likely etiology for the lesions. Cryptococcosis, streptococcal pharyngitis, and tuberculosis are also associated with erythema nodosum, but the symptomatology does not support these diagnoses. Thus, the best test on the list is barium enema, although some might prefer colonoscopy. A chest X-ray would be helpful to look for evidence of cryptococcal or tuberculous infection, and a throat culture might identify Group A streptococci. A Tine test would be entirely reasonable.

Further Discussion

The lesions of erythema nodosum appear as deep, tender nodules on the extensor surfaces of the extremities. Palpation helps to make the diagnosis, as one can best appreciate the depth of the lesions by touch. Erythema nodosum occurs as a hypersensitivity reaction to a number of underlying diseases or exposures. In my experience, the most common precipitant is the use of oral contraceptives in an adolescent female. Next in frequency is streptococcal pharyngitis. In selected geographic areas, histoplasmosis and other systemic fungal infections should receive prominent consideration. Of the chronic underlying conditions, inflammatory bowel disease is most likely. Other considerations include tuberculosis, sarcoidosis, and rarely malignancies.

A father brings in his 7-year-old son in due to groin pain and limp. The father noted the limp today, but the boy says that his groin has been painful for "a long time."

1. After viewing the radiograph you ask the father whether his son:
   A. Has been in any accidents recently?
   B. Has had any fevers in the last few weeks?
   C. Has ever taken corticosteroids?
   D. Has had any other joint pains or swelling?
   E. Has had a rubella immunization recently?

2. Treatment for this problem includes:
   A. Oral cephalexin
   B. Joint aspiration
   C. Intravenous oxacillin
   D. Surgery
   E. Prednisone

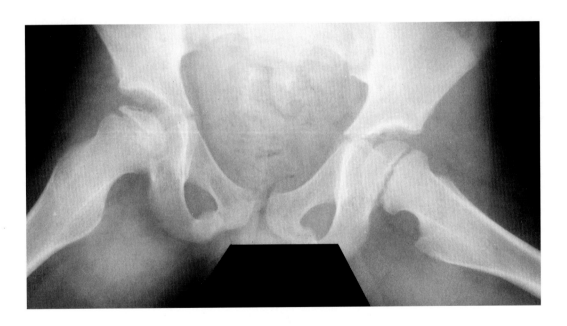

DISCUSSION

ANSWERS:

1. **C. Has ever taken corticosteroids?**
2. **D. Surgery**

1. The radiograph does not indicate any acute or old fractures or avulsions or show any signs of osteomyelitis or a hip effusion, making trauma and infection unlikely. Additionally, absence of a joint effusion speaks against toxic synovitis, juvenile rheumatoid arthritis, rheumatic fever, or post-rubella immunization synovitis. The right femoral head is small and flattened, suggesting an avascular necrosis syndrome. Avascular necrosis of the femoral head can be found in patients who have taken corticosteroids.

2. Since no joint effusion exists, a joint aspiration is not indicated. Neither oral nor intravenous antimicrobials are useful for avascular necrosis. Prednisone is contraindicated in patients with avascular necrosis syndromes. The treatment of avascular necrosis syndromes like Legg-Calve-Perthes (LCP) disease may consist of observation, bed rest, braces, casts, or surgery to prevent progressive deformity of the femoral head and degenerative arthritis.

Further Discussion

LCP disease or avascular necrosis of the femoral head is caused by interruption of the blood supply to the femoral head. Patients with LCP disease are usually Caucasian males between 4 and 8 years of age and often fall below average for height and weight. Patients present with symptoms much like this child or may have predominant knee or thigh complaints or even a painless limp. Avascular necrosis may cause limited motion of the hip, especially internal rotation and abduction. The anterior hip may be tender. The diagnosis can be delayed since early radiographs may be normal. Other causes of avascular necrosis, such as sickle cell anemia, Gaucher's disease, and corticosteroid use, need to be ruled out.

A 6-week-old infant arrives in the emergency department by ambulance. The medics were called to the home to pick up this baby, whose mother reported persisted vomiting for about a week followed by the onset of lethargy over the last 24 hours. In the emergency department, the child is pale and lifeless. Vital signs are: P 210/min, R 38/min, BP 70/40 mm Hg, and T 38.1°C. The positive findings are shown. You initiate resuscitation with normal saline at 20 cc/kg.

1. The test most likely to lead to a diagnosis is:
    A. Intravenous pyelogram
    B. Retrograde urethrogram
    C. Upper gastrointestinal series
    D. Urinary steroid measurement
    E. Lumbar puncture

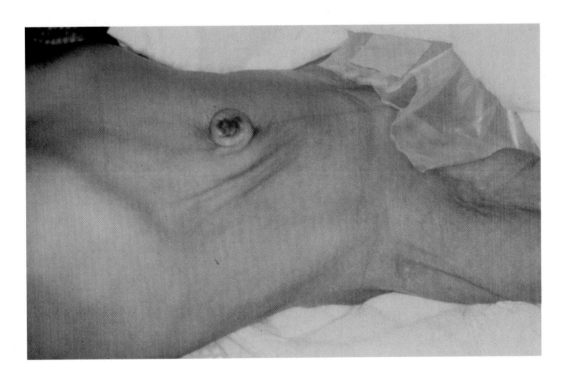

DISCUSSION

ANSWER:

1. C. **Upper gastrointestinal series**

1. Tenting of the skin indicates that this child has marked dehydration and the vital signs suggest circulatory failure resulting from volume loss; in combination with a scaphoid abdomen, these findings point to pyloric stenosis, which may be diagnosed either by abdominal ultrasound or by an upper gastrointestinal series. Posterior urethral valves may cause hydronephrosis, electrolyte disturbances and dehydration, usually with a distended abdomen; the diagnosis is established by retrograde urethrogram. Hirschsprung's disease is also likely to result in marked abdominal distension. Diagnosis of Hirschsprung's disease often relies on rectal manometry or biopsy, but a barium enema may be helpful. Congenital adrenal hyperplasia (CAH) of the salt losing variety may present with acute onset of dehydration and shock, but not necessarily with a scaphoid abdomen. Females with CAH may have ambiguous genitalia. This condition results from a metabolic disorder affecting the adrenal glands and leads to an abnormal pattern of urinary steroid excretion. Meningitis may produce persistent vomiting, but one would expect a shorter course and a history of fever.

Further Discussion

Once a patient is stabilized, the physician must sometimes play the odds in staging a diagnostic work-up. In this case, the physical examination yielded no pathognomonic signs and all the disorders listed, being reasonable elements of the differential diagnosis, might be pursued. However, given that pyloric stenosis is far and away the most common cause of persistent vomiting in a child this age with this examination, it makes sense to search for it first. Failure to palpate an "olive" should not dissuade the clinician, as absence of a mass does not rule out the diagnosis. The likelihood of successful palpation may be enhanced by emptying the stomach with a nasogastric tube and by holding the infant's legs off the examining table.

CASE 80

A 9-year-old comes into the emergency department with acute onset of rash on his left chest and back. The lesions erupted 3 days ago and have spread. He has been generally well and afebrile.

1. Based on the findings you would:
   A. Start acyclovir intravenously
   B. Prescribe acyclovir topically
   C. Give oral antibiotics
   D. Recommend aspirin for fever
   E. None of the above

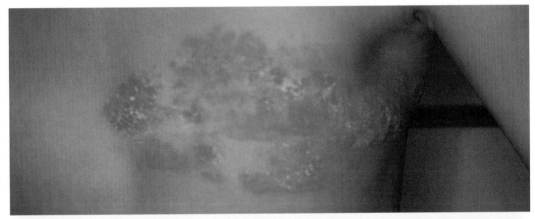

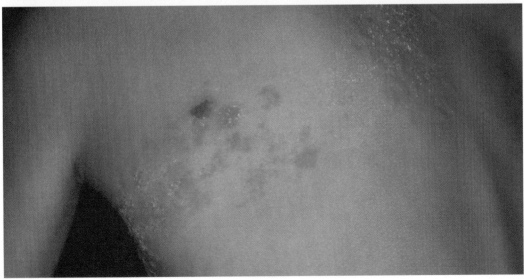

DISCUSSION

ANSWER:

1. E. None of the above

1. The correct action is to do none of the above. The lesions are diagnostic of herpes zoster. The only treatment that may be needed is symptomatic therapy for pain and pruritis, as the eruption will resolve spontaneously. Aspirin, however, is contraindicated due to the association between aspirin use in patients with varicella and Reye syndrome.

Further Discussion

Herpes zoster or shingles is a manifestation of varicilla-zoster virus, which occurs as a result of reactivation of a latent, persistent infection. It appears as a papulovesicular eruption in a sensory nerve distribution. This condition is not usually painful in children, as it is in adults. It is also not associated with underlying neoplastic disease, so patients do not need to be evaluated for occult malignancy. Acyclovir intravenously should be used only if the patient is an immunocompromised host.

Some sources state that zoster is rare in children, but this is emphatically not the case. Although the eruption follows primary varicella by a number of years, it is seen in children of all ages, particularly among those with varicella early in life. The only situation where zoster occurs in a patient without prior varicella is among children who have been exposed during gestation, prior to the last week or so of pregnancy.

Unlike chickenpox, which is transmitted by respiratory droplets, the open lesions of zoster are the major source of spread. Health care personnel and others who have not had chickenpox will need to be protected.

A 10-month-old is brought to the emergency department with fever and an area of redness and induration on the cheek. The child is reported to be otherwise well. She has received no prior health care as her parents do not have any health insurance. On examination the child is in no acute distress and has a temperature of 38.8°C. She appears uncomfortable when you palpate the lesion shown below.

1. Based on your examination you conclude the most likely diagnosis is:
   A. "Popsicle" panniculitis
   B. Facial cellulitis
   C. A contusion
   D. A dental abscess
   E. Fifth disease

2. In order to solidify the diagnosis you should:
   A. Obtain a CT of the orbits
   B. Obtain a complete blood count
   C. Obtain dental x-rays
   D. Measure parvovirus antibody titers
   E. Obtain more history

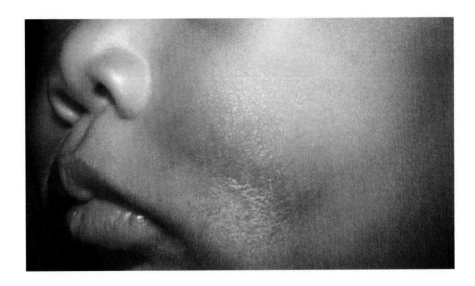

DISCUSSION

ANSWERS:
1. **B. Facial cellulitis**
2. **B. Obtain a complete blood count**

1. This is a case of facial cellulitis. Cold ("popsicle") panniculitis may have a very similar appearance in a child who is otherwise asymptomatic and afebrile with a mildly tender lesion. A history of cold exposure is very important in making the diagnosis; this might be a popsicle or the application of ice to the cheek by parents to treat irritability from the eruption of new teeth. A dental abscess may produce painful swelling of the cheek, but it would be an unusual diagnosis at this age, as most children only have a few anterior teeth at 10 months. Fifth disease, an infection with parvovirus, produces a "slapped cheek" appearance, but it is bilateral, superficial, and nontender. It lacks the induration noted in this case. A low grade fever and upper respiratory symptoms are also usual features in Fifth disease. Trauma is always a possible diagnosis. History is usually helpful, but if the trauma was inflicted, the parents may conceal the story. A traumatic injury changes over the first 24 hours and the lesion appears to spread out, as blood layers in a fascial plane. Traumatic injury usually takes on a blue hue, and trauma does not usually produce a febrile response.

2. The total white blood cell count is useful in children with facial cellulitis, as it is often elevated in response to the infection, particularly when there is an accompanying bacteremia. A CT scan would be helpful in differentiating orbital from periorbital cellulitis, but is not indicated in buccal lesions. For an older child with a similar picture, particularly with the finding of carious teeth, dental X-rays would be appropriate. Although a detailed history is always advisable, it is unlikely to provide any further clues in this case.

Further Discussion

Facial cellulitis is one of a number of diseases seen less often with the use of the *Hemophilus influenzae* vaccine. Like meningitis, epiglottitis and other *H. influenzae* infections, the incidence has decreased markedly in the United States since 1995. Other organisms such as group A streptococci, *Streptococcus pneumoniae*, and *Staphylococcus aureus* have been reported to produce identical findings.

The mother of this 3-month girl seeks care at 1 a.m. for a "rash" on her daughter's chin. She noticed the lesions for the first time 1 hour ago. The baby has been in good health, but according to the mother missed her immunizations at 2 months of age because she had a "cold." On examination, the child is vigorous and in no distress. Her temperature is 37.3°C. You palpate her liver and spleen 1 cm below the costal margins. Otherwise, her physical examination is unremarkable.

1. Your next step would be to:
   A. Order an RPR
   B. Obtain a social work evaluation
   C. Administer intramuscular benzathine penicillin
   D. Consult a dermatologist
   E. Prescribe erythromycin

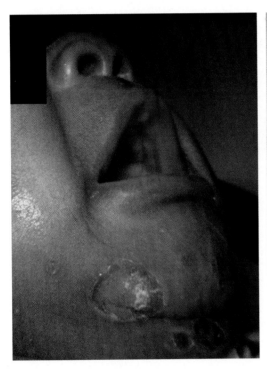
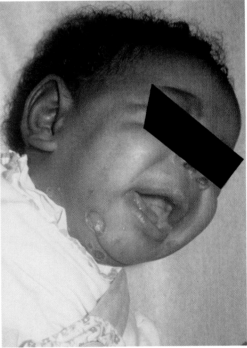

DISCUSSION

ANSWER:

1. E. Prescribe erythromycin

1. This little girl has bullous impetigo. When the bullae slough off, as has happened here, the lesions may resemble cigarette burns, at times intentionally inflicted as a form of child abuse. The varying size of the lesions and the crusted, rather than erythematous appearance, point toward impetigo in this case. Secondary syphilis affects the labial commissures, but not the chin. While it would never be inappropriate in a clinical setting to consult either a dermatologist or a social worker if you were uncertain about a case, the lesions here are sufficiently typical that most physicians would be comfortable treating for impetigo. *S. aureus* causes a greater proportion of impetigo than *S. pyogenes* in recent years, particularly when the morphology is bullous. Thus, erythromycin is the best choice. Although benzathine penicillin is recommended in some older texts for impetigo that is not bullous, I do not use this drug routinely anymore, as a result of the increased prevalence of *S. aureus*.

A 15-year-old comes to the emergency department with complaints of tiring while playing basketball. This has been progressive over the past 4 weeks. He mentions no other symptoms. His chest wall appears normal and is nontender. Examination of his heart reveals no murmurs, rubs, or gallops.

1. Initial therapy might include:
   A. Atropine
   B. Epinephrine
   C. Isoproterenol
   D. Pacemaker
   E. None of the above

2. What is the cause for this problem?
   A. Systemic lupus erythematosus
   B. Myocardial infarction
   C. Prior surgical repair of congenital heart disease
   D. Myocarditis
   E. Transposition of the great arteries

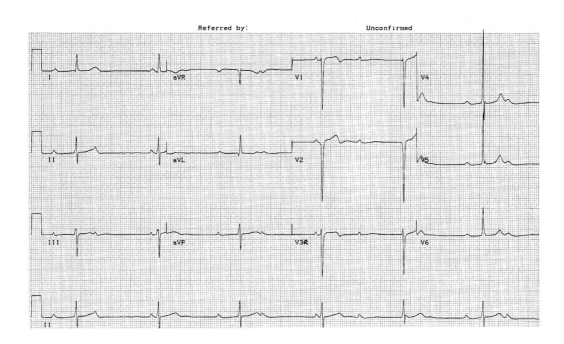

DISCUSSION

ANSWERS:
1. E. None of the above
2. D. Myocarditis

1. Although the patient is bradycardic, he does not have chest pain, acute shortness of breath, decreased level of consciousness, shock, or congestive heart failure. No immediate therapy is needed. In the hemodynamically stable patient, standard guidelines do not call for atropine, epinephrine or immediate insertion of a pacemaker.

2. The tracing shows a ventricular rate of 36/min, without a consistent relationship between the P wave and the QRS complex. This is complete heart block. There is some variation in the sinus rate. The QRS width is .08 indicating a fairly high escape rhythm (i.e., in or above the His bundle). The most common cause of congenital complete heart block in infants is autoimmune injury to the conduction system by maternal IgG antibodies from a mother with systemic lupus erythematosus, but these children present as neonates or within the first few months of life. Complete heart block may develop after an acute myocardial infarction; however, this patient has no evidence of such as event. The most common cause of acquired complete heart block in children is prior surgical repair of congenital heart disease involving the ventricular septum. Since the patient lacks a scar on his chest, this is unlikely. Complete heart block may be acquired after myocarditis, even when subclinical, or with the development of a myocardial tumor. Complete heart block may be seen with structural heart disease like L-transposition of the great arteries, but it is unlikely that a teenage patient with uncorrected transposition of the great arteries would have no prior history of cardiac problems.

A 10-day-old infant developed a lesion in her left breast 2 days ago. The swelling has increased and today the area appears erythematous. The father reports that the baby has been taking her bottle well and that her temperature on two occasions was 37°C. Currently, she is afebrile and generally appears well.

1. Your recommendation to the father for treatment is:
    A. Incision and drainage
    B. Oral cephalexin
    C. Observation
    D. Intravenous gentamicin
    E. Lupron®

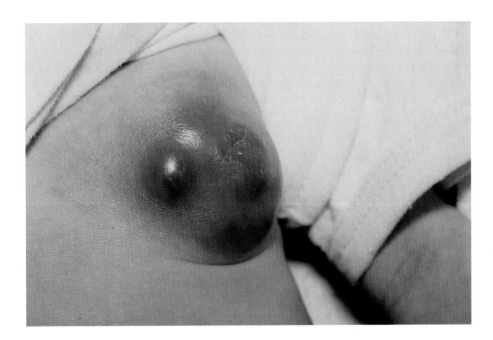

DISCUSSION

ANSWER:

1. A. Incision and drainage

1. Unlike an earlier patient with physiologic gynecomastia and "witches' milk" (see Case 32), this infant has a mastitis that has developed an area of fluctuance. The primary treatment, as there is an obvious abscess, is incision and drainage. Additionally, I would start intravenous oxacillin (or another antistaphylococcal antibiotic) and gentamicin. *Staphylococcal aureus* causes the majority of neonatal mastitis, with gram-negative enteric rods in second place but trailing far behind. An oral cephalosporin, such as cephalexin, possesses excellent activity against *S. aureus* but lacks sufficiently potency in a deep soft tissue infection of the newborn with the potential for bacteremia. Lupron® is a luteinizing hormone antagonist that has no role here.

Further Discussion

Mastitis occurs at the extremes of the pediatric age range, in neonates (either male or female) and in adolescents (female). Stimulation of the breast tissue in the neonate by transplacentally passed maternal hormones creates a local anatomic milieu similar to that seen in the teenage female. Under these conditions, bacteremia may ascend along the ducts in the glandular tissue of the breast and establish an infection. Most cases of mastitis can be treated successfully with intravenous antibiotics, avoiding the need for surgical intervention. Since incision may potentially damage the underlying breast bud, it must be done extremely carefully, particularly in females, to avoid later cosmetic deformity.

An 8-month child with recurrent previously diagnosed neutropenia of unknown etiology has had a fever for 3 days. She was evaluated for fever and cough at another facility 24 hours earlier, where her WBC count was 7,200/ mm^3 (60% neutrophils) and her chest X-ray was normal. Since that time, she has become progressively more lethargic. Her past history is remarkable for a "malignant" otitis externa at the age of 3 months, caused by *Pseudomonas aeruginosa.*

Vital signs:	P 174/min R 28/min BP 65/45 mm Hg T 39.1°C
General	Pale, gray
HEENT	Pharynx without injection
Nodes	No adenopathy
Neck	Supple
Lungs	No rales or wheezes
Heart	No murmurs, quiet precordium, faint pulses
Abdomen	Mild tenderness; liver palpable 2 cm below the right costal margin
Neurologic	Lethargic with no focal findings

1. The nurse is administering 100% oxygen and two of your colleagues have set off in pursuit of intravenous access. Your next step in treatment is:
   A. Air enema
   B. Pericardiocentesis
   C. Ceftriaxone intravenously
   D. Dopamine intravenously
   E. Chest tube insertion

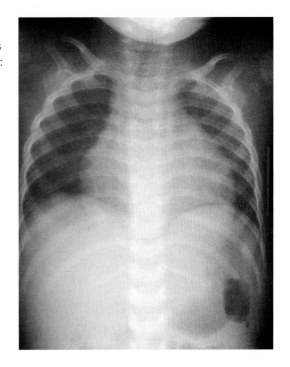

DISCUSSION

ANSWER:

1. **B. Pericardiocentesis**

1. In this child, who has experienced rapid onset of profound shock 3 days into a febrile illness, cardiomegaly on X-ray is the most striking finding. She has no history of congenital heart disease and you have not auscultated a murmur, so congestive failure on the basis of a structural abnormality is unlikely. Aberrant coronary arteries may cause shock and cardiomegaly, but the onset of this clinical syndrome usually occurs at 3 to 4 months of age and would not generally be preceded by a fever. More likely possibilities include myocarditis and pericarditis. The fever, abrupt increase in heart size over 24 hours, and susceptibility to bacterial infections in this child with a neutrophil abnormality, taken together, point to purulent pericarditis with tamponade. Thus, the next therapeutic step is pericardiocentesis after a stat echocardiogram, if time allows. If you suspected myocarditis, infusion of dopamine to support the circulation along with other measures to treat her shock is a reasonable choice. Intussusception peaks at 5 to10 months of age and may lead to shock and obtundation due to third spacing of fluids and the production of cytokines; air contrast enema for reduction, and of course for diagnosis, is the optimal modality to deal with this entity. A chest tube would correct a tension pneumothorax, but one is not present here; there is neither air in the pleural space nor a shift of the mediastinum. The administration of ceftriaxone for generalized sepsis or purulent pericarditis is most appropriate, but should not delay the drainage of the pus from the pericardial sac.

CASE 86

The frantic parents of a 2-week-old infant rush into the emergency department in the late afternoon because, just minutes before their arrival, they noticed a rash on their baby's abdomen. The mother reports that the child, born at term by spontaneous vaginal delivery after an uncomplicated pregnancy, had been thriving and earlier in the day had a normal checkup at her doctor's office. The infant is afebrile and appears vigorous.

1. Your diagnosis is:
   A. Thermal injury
   B. Ichthyosis
   C. Omphalitis
   D. Chemical burn
   E. Scalded skin syndrome

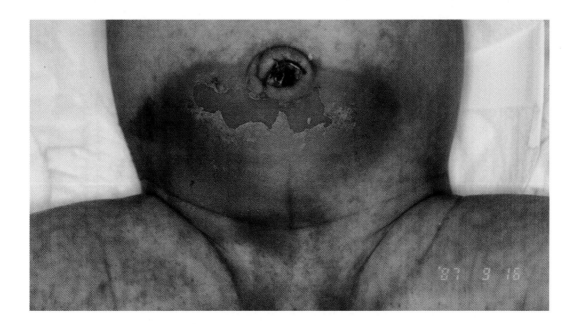

DISCUSSION

ANSWER:

1. D. Chemical burn

1. This is a chemical burn. No, it is not secondary to either an environmental disaster or child abuse, but rather to an iatrogenic mishap. Earlier in this book, you diagnosed an umbilical granuloma (see Case 60) and recommended the topical application of silver nitrate. I hope that you had in mind to apply the silver nitrate sparingly, taking care to avoid the surrounding skin and to cover the umbilicus afterwards to prevent weeping. Six hours after leaving his pediatrician's office, this infant came to the emergency department as pictured.

Further Discussion

Silver nitrate is useful for cauterizing various lesions, but it has the potential to cause serious injury, particularly to the skin of an infant. In this case, grafting was needed to repair the defect created, when the damaged tissues of the anterior abdominal wall sloughed.

A 13-year-old male complains of pain surrounding his hip. At basketball practice, while running for a lay-up, he heard a "pop" which was followed by excruciating pain and inability to bear weight. On physical examination there is no obvious swelling or ecchymosis. He guards his hip, yet has no direct tenderness over the hip joint. An X-ray of his hip is shown.

1. Appropriate management of this patient is:
    A. Immediate orthopedic consultation
    B. Bed rest for 4 weeks
    C. Anti-inflammatory medication and crutches
    D. Orthopedic consultation with intraoperative fixation
    E. Pelvic CT scan to further delineate the injury

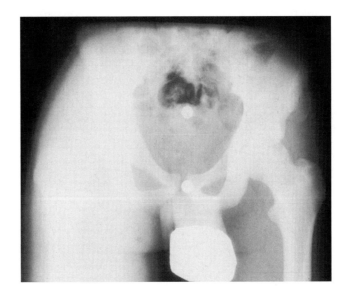

DISCUSSION

ANSWERS:

1. **C. Anti-inflammatory medication and crutches**

1. The anterior iliac physis is one of the last to close and is the insertion site for the sartorius muscle. Avulsion injuries at this site are not unusual among adolescents who have large, well-developed hip flexors. Most patients have an acute episode of pain that interrupts activity. There is point tenderness over the anterior iliac spine, and movement of the lower extremity results in tremendous pain as the avulsed fragment is moved. Usually, there is incomplete separation. In this example, however, displacement of the avulsed fracture fragment is easily seen. Conservative treatment with non-weight bearing, pain management and outpatient orthopedic follow-up is indicated. Athletic activities should be avoided for a period of 4 to 6 weeks. Complications are rare.

Further Discussion

Surprisingly, even displaced fractures respond to a brief period of bed rest and subsequent guarded weight bearing on crutches for 2 weeks. In a series of nine patients, all seven treated with this conservative fashion healed with full recovery of hip function.

A 15-month-old is brought in with a painful swollen finger. The child is afebrile and has no other apparent physical findings. The mother reports that the child sucks his fingers. She sought medical attention for this 2 days ago and was given a prescription for antibiotics. There has been no improvement, and the finger is shown below.

1. As you assess the situation you conclude that the cause is:
   A. Local trauma
   B. A bacterial infection
   C. Immune deficiency
   D. A viral infection
   E. An insect bite

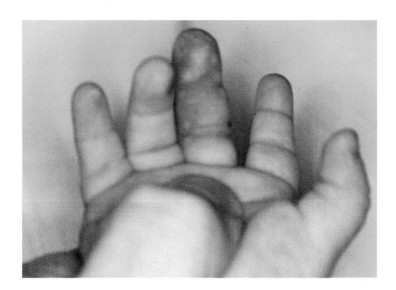

DISCUSSION

ANSWERS:

1. **D. A viral infection**

1. This is another example of herpetic whitlow (see Case 37), demonstrating that some children suck their fingers instead of their thumbs. Careful inspection shows 4-6 separate vesicular lesions. They involve only the finger and have not spread in a wider distribution, as one might see with herpes zoster. The most likely cause is Herpes simplex type 1; the original lesions may have been in the patient's mouth, but are no longer visible. The lesions may have also been contacted from another child. One does not need to postulate an immune deficiency, as this infection strikes otherwise healthy children. Grouped vesicular lesions are rarely caused by bacteria, as is seen in the entity known as blistering distal dactylitis, usually due to streptococci. Both a Gram stain and a Tzanck preparation may be helpful in differentiating between viral and bacterial infections on the spot, but cultures are best for a definitive diagnosis. Local trauma and insect bites are possible reasons for swelling and erythema of a digit, but they do not generally produce multiple, grouped vesicular lesions.

Further Discussion

Although we usually think of herpetic disease in immunocompetent hosts as being confined to the oral and genital regions, this is not necessarily the case. Intact skin acts as a barrier to infection, but the virus will take advantage of any breaks in the integument. Herpetic whitlow presumably results from penetration in an area where moisture and friction have caused the skin to break down. Herpetic infections also occur over the extensor surfaces of joints in wrestlers (herpes gladiatorum) and in burned areas.

This severely dehydrated infant has in place both an intraosseous needle and a catheter inserted using the cutdown technique.

1. The site chosen for the cutdown incision was:
   A. 1 cm inferior to the medial malleolus
   B. Immediately posterior to the medial malleolus
   C. Immediately superior to the medial malleolus
   D. 1 cm anterior to the medial malleolus
   E. Directly over the medial malleolus

2. The vein that has been cannulated is the:
   A. Lesser saphenous
   B. Posterior tibial
   C. Lesser popliteal
   D. Anterior tibial
   E. Inferior gluteal

3. A potential complication from the intraosseous infusion is:
   A. Aplastic anemia
   B. Septic arthritis
   C. Hemolytic anemia
   D. Fat necrosis
   E. Compartment syndrome

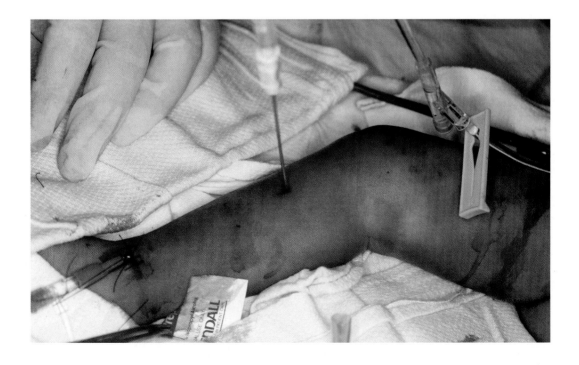

DISCUSSION

ANSWERS:

1. **D. 1 cm anterior to the medial malleolus**
2. **A. Lesser saphenous**
3. **E. Compartment syndrome**

1. The incision for a cutdown at the ankle is 1 cm anterior to the medial malleolus.

2. The vein being cannulated is the lesser saphenous. If time allows, the vein is located by gently spreading the tissues, using a curved hemostat. In more urgent situations, all the tissues anterior to the malleolus can be picked up at once with the tip of the hemostat. Once the vessel is isolated, two ligatures are placed under it. Traditionally, the distal ligature is tied, an incision is made into the vein, a catheter is advanced through the incision, and the proximal ligature is tied. Alternatively, as in this case, the distal ligature can be left untied but used for traction and a catheter-over-the-needle device advanced into the vein.

3. Intraosseous infusions rarely lead to complications, but several recent reports have noted compartment syndrome following infiltration. Fat embolism, of uncertain significance, and osteomyelitis are also described. Septic arthritis should not occur, unless a joint space is entered inadvertently. Injury to the hematopoietic cells has not been reported.

Further Discussion

Venous access, always challenging in young infants, may be life-saving in many situations. To increase the likelihood of a successful outcome, physicians should have a game plan laid out to deal with critically ill patients. The exact procedures and sequencing will vary. In this infant, when peripheral venous cannulation proved too time consuming, an intraosseous needle was placed. Because intraosseous access provides only a temporary solution, a more definitive solution was achieved with a saphenous cutdown. Percutaneous catheterization of the femoral vein, using a guidewire, would have been a reasonable alternative.

A 16-year-old male comes to the emergency department complaining of severe scrotal pain. The pain started at 7:30 PM the previous day and, when it persisted, he came to the emergency department. He gives a history of sexual activity 1 week ago and bumping into a table 3 days prior. His vital signs are as follows: P 120/min, R 18/min, BP 140/80 mm Hg, and T 37.2°C. His examination is normal except for a right horizontal testis as noted below.

1. Based on these findings you would diagnose:
   A. Epididymitis
   B. Torsion of the appendix testis
   C. Torsion of the testis
   D. Varicocele
   E. Testicular tumor

2. The best way to confirm the diagnosis is:
   A. Urinalysis
   B. Urethral culture
   C. Doppler ultrasound
   D. Radionuclide scan
   E. Surgical exploration

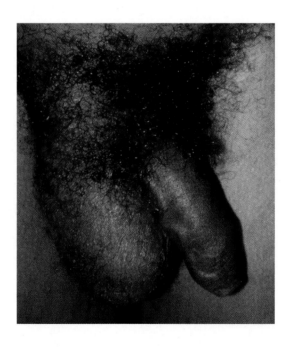

DISCUSSION

ANSWERS:
1. C. Torsion of the testis
2. E. Surgical exploration

1. The findings point to torsion of the testis, as this boy has a swollen hemiscrotum and a testis that is elevated in the scrotum in a horizontal lie (i.e., long axis of the testis in the horizontal plane). The elements in the story that further support the diagnosis include both the abrupt onset and severity of the pain, such that the vital signs are altered. Neither the history of sexual activity nor the report of minor trauma should dissuade one from pursuing the most serious diagnosis, that of torsion. In some cases, minor trauma to the scrotum, or even trauma to a nearby area, may be the trigger for the torsion. Epididymitis may cause similar swelling to the testicle, but the history should be of a more gradual onset and the testicular lie would be normal. Other findings that may help to differentiate epididymitis from torsion of the testis include the presence of a cremasteric reflex and the relief of the pain with manual elevation of the testis in patients with epididymitis. Torsion of the appendix testis may produce scrotal pain, but it is usually localized to one point. Generally, the pain is not as severe as in torsion, and the position of the testicle in the scrotum is normal. Particularly in prepubertal children, but also in teenagers with findings compatible with torsion of the testis, epididymitis and torsion of the appendix testis are considered diagnoses of exclusion; ruling out torsion must be the first priority. Varicocele produces a "bag of worms" appearance of the scrotum. Although this condition does cause mild discomfort, it does not produce the extreme pain of testicular torsion. Additionally, varicocele almost always affects the left testis.

2. Although Doppler testing and radionuclide scans would support the clinical diagnosis, the signs are sufficiently distinct in this case that the most appropriate course is to refer the patient to a surgeon for exploration and repair. The other methods of detection each have their shortcomings and should not be relied upon to exclude torsion in a case when the clinical findings are strongly suggestive. Doppler ultrasound and radionuclide scanning primarily serve to substantiate the absence of testicular torsion in a case where the prior probability, based on clinical evaluation, is low. With epididymitis, both a urinalysis, showing pyuria, and a urethral culture, particularly for gonorrhea, may be helpful

Further Discussion

One needs to keep in mind that the symptoms of torsion may change over time. The pain may diminish, if the testis becomes infarcted and dies. Thus, on day two of the process, the pain may be less. Furthermore, some teenagers may be extremely stoic. Do not be fooled!

A precocious 2-year-old boy falls onto outstretched hands while jumping on the couch at the obstetrician's office, as his mother waits for her appointment. The child grabs the left side of his neck and screams with pain, refusing to move. An EMT arrives, straps him onto a posterior spine board, and brings him to the emergency department. He lies comfortably immobilized and has no neurologic deficits on your examination. As soon as you open his collar, he screams with pain and grabs the left side of his neck.

1. Which of the following tests would be most helpful?
    A. Lateral cervical spine X-ray
    B. Lateral, anteroposterior and odontoid cervical spine X-rays
    C. A CT scan of the upper cervical spine
    D. An MRI of the cervical spine
    E. Clavicle X-rays

DISCUSSION

ANSWERS:

1. **E. Clavicle X-rays**

1. Always remember to consider the mechanism of injury in conjunction with the physical examination. This child experienced a low energy impact and was described to have fallen on an outstretched hand, making a clavicular fracture the most likely injury. Simply palpating along the shaft of this bone might help in deciding on the most appropriate X-ray. Although a fracture or dislocation of the cervical spine is possible, injuries of this type are rare in children after minor trauma. While one could not be faulted for obtaining cervical spine X-rays, neither a CT scan nor an MRI make any sense at this point.

Further Discussion

The clavicle is the most common bone fractured in children. Fractures usually occur after falls on an outstretched hand, falls onto the shoulder, or direct blows to the clavicle. Patients may present with pain, swelling and tenderness at the site of the fracture, with torticollis due to neck pain, as the sternocleidomastoid muscles insert on the clavicle, or with pseudoparalysis of the upper extremity. The vast majority of clavicular fractures occur in the midshaft, with less than 10% occurring at the medial or distal ends. They are most typically greenstick fractures or plastic deformations, and in many cases a clear fracture line is not readily visible. In viewing the X-rays, it is important to note patient position, as rotation can make the normal bowing of the clavicle appear abnormal. Remember that, since plastic bowing and greenstick fractures occur commonly, abnormal shape of the clavicle in the proper clinical setting should be treated as a fracture. Since the periosteum is so strong in young children, it prevents significant displacement of the fracture fragments making neurovascular injury rare, despite the proximity of these structure as they course behind the clavicle. Medial fractures usually involve the epiphysis, and posterior or anterior displacement may occur. Distal fractures also usually occur at the physis. Upward displacement of the distal fragment is often seen with distal fractures as the periosteum remains attached to the ligaments of the acromio-clavicular joint.

Clavicle fractures heal rapidly due to the presence of intact periosteum. Immobilization with a figure-of-eight bandage, clavicle strap, or a sling is recommended to prevent further displacement and to minimize pain. This should be worn for 3 weeks, and contact sports should be avoided for an additional 3 weeks. Warn the parents that the healing bone will result in an unsightly lump that will naturally remodel over the year following the injury. Orthopedic consultation is rarely necessary and is helpful primarily when sterno-clavicular dislocation occurs.

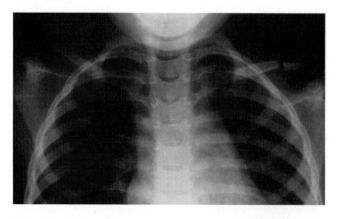

The mother of a 10-year-old girl is concerned that she may have been abused. The parents are divorced and the girl stayed with her father and his girlfriend for 2 months over the summer. When the youngster returned, she complained to her mother of a rash. Despite intensive questioning by her mother, she denied that anyone had abused her in any fashion. She has been previously healthy. On examination, she appears well and is afebrile.

1. As you prepare to perform the rest of the examination, you expect to find:
   A. Bruises of varying age
   B. Scaling behind the ears
   C. Lichenification of the antecubital fossae
   D. Small perianal worms
   E. None of the above

2. After completing your assessment, you would:
   A. Prescribe mebendazole orally
   B. Make a report of suspected child abuse
   C. Request a gynecologic exam under anesthesia
   D. Refer the family for a social service evaluation
   E. Recommend a steroid cream

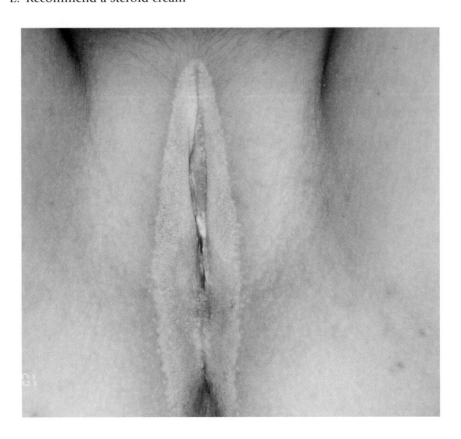

DISCUSSION

ANSWERS:

1. E. None of the above
2. E. Recommend a steroid cream

1. This girl has lichen sclerosis et atrophicus, so none of the options are correct. Bruises of varying age may be a sign of physical abuse, which is not the correct diagnosis here. Even if you did incorrectly suspect sexual abuse in this girl, keep in mind that accompanying physical injury is rare in children. Seborrhea may cause a rash in the posterior auricular area, but not lesions of the labia. Similarly, atopic dermatitis or eczema may manifest with lichenification of the antecubital fossae in children of this age, but generally does not involve the genitalia. Pinworms may affect the vagina as well as the anus; pruritus without rash is the most frequent manifestation.

2. Topical steroids provide some help with lichen sclerosis et atrophicus. In our society, any lesion close to the genitals raises the specter of sexual abuse and may engender unnecessary evaluations and reports. This is true for lichen sclerosis. However, one should be able to make this diagnosis with certainty based on the morphology and distribution of the rash, thereby obviating the need to involve social service agencies. Oral mebendazole is recommended for pinworms.

Further Discussion

Lichen sclerosus et atrophicus (more recently referred to simply as lichen sclerosis) is more common in older women, but does occur in prepubertal girls. It typically manifests with depigmentation in an "hourglass" distribution. The cause of this disorder has not been identified.

A 5-week-old infant is referred to you for evaluation of cardiomegaly. He presented to an outlying emergency department with one day of irritability and upper respiratory infection symptoms. During his evaluation, a chest radiograph was obtained. On physical examination, he is well-appearing, with a heart rate of 145/min, a blood pressure of 70/45 mm Hg and a respiratory rate of 40/min. His room air pulse oximeter reading is 98%. He has no murmur, no pulmonary findings, and no organomegaly.

1. You accept him for transfer, and suspect that his most likely diagnosis is:
   A. Ventricular septal defect
   B. Congenital cardiomyopathy
   C. Normal infant
   D. Mediastinal tumor
   E. Pneumonia

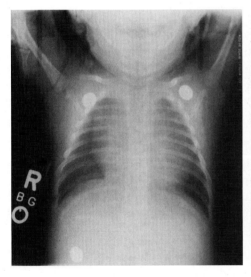 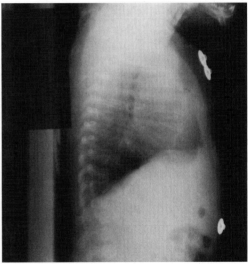

DISCUSSION

ANSWER:

1. C. Normal infant

1. In reviewing this baby's X-ray, the widened mediastinum is attributable to normal thymus. The base of the heart appears to be of normal width, and the lateral view reveals no prominence of the ventricle pushing posteriorly on the airway. Further, the child is well with a normal physical examination. This is a normal chest radiograph in an infant. The thymus has an extremely variable appearance on the chest radiograph, changing considerably with inspiration and expiration. It lies anterior to the great vessels and covers the top portion of the heart in an umbrella-like fashion. Although present up to puberty, it is usually not apparent on the chest radiograph beyond the ages of 2 to 3 years. Look for the "sail sign" of the right lobe as it overlies the heart. Also, look for scalloped borders that help in distinguishing thymus from cardiac shadow. Occasionally, it is difficult to distinguish cardiomegaly from the thymic shadow. The lateral X-ray is helpful in such a scenario as with true cardiomegaly the margin of the left ventricle is displaced posteriorly. The thymic shadow also may be misinterpreted as upper lobe pneumonia or mediastinal mass. Again, look for the smooth, wavy borders of the thymus and look at the lateral X-ray.

Further Discussion

When reviewing X-rays of older children, adolescents and adults, the heart size is evaluated using the cardiothoracic ratio. Drop two vertical lines tangential to the most prominent points on the right and left heart borders and measure the distance between them. This width should be less than half the widest intra-thoracic diameter, measured from the inner aspect of the rib cage at its widest point. Limiting factors in obtaining accurate measurement include radiologic technique, degree of patient inspiration, chest wall deformities, scoliosis, or abdominal distension.

In infants and small children, measurement of the cardiothoracic ratio is less helpful. Remember that most infants have anteroposterior radiographs done while in the supine position with variable degrees of inspiration and rotation. Additionally, infants have compliant chest walls and mediastinal structures, in addition to large abdomens. All of these factors obviously affect the accuracy with which measurements can be made.

A 6-year-old boy complains of swelling in his axilla for 3 days. He does not mention a sore throat. Although his father thinks he felt warm on several occasions, no measurement of his temperature has been documented. He has not experienced any decrease in his appetite or weight loss, but has been fatigued.

On examination, his temperature is 37.9°C orally. He appears generally well and has a clear pharynx. Minimal, shoddy, anterior cervical adenopathy is present bilaterally. Neither the liver nor the spleen is palpable.

1. The etiology for this boy's problem is:
   A. *Rochalimea (Bartonella) hensleae*
   B. Cytomegalovirus
   C. Epstein Barr virus
   D. Group A *Streptococcus*
   E. *Toxoplasmosis gondii*

2. He is at risk for:
   A. Splenic rupture
   B. Retinitis
   C. Liver failure
   D. Encephalitis
   E. Peritonsillar abscess

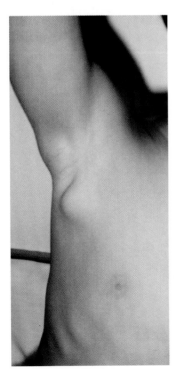
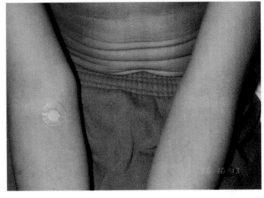

DISCUSSION

ANSWERS:
1. A. *Rochalimea (Bartonella) hensleae*
2. D. **Encephalitis**

1. This boy has two enlarged lymph nodes, one in the right axilla and the other in the right epitrochlear area. He is afebrile and does not have posterior cervical adenopathy, pharyngitis, or hepatosplenomegaly. When acute, isolated lymph node enlargement without systemic illness is usually the result of an infection in a contiguous structure (reactive adenopathy) or in the node (adenitis). The most common cause of adenitis is infection with either *Staphylococcus aureus* or *Streptococcus pyogenes*, followed by *Rochalimea hensleae* (cat scratch disease) and atypical mycobacteria. Both the distribution of the nodes (epitrochlear and axillary) and the relatively quiet appearance point to cat scratch disease. Further down on the left arm, the boy had several healing abrasions; more focused questioning revealed the purchase of a kitten 6 months earlier.

2. Patients with cat scratch disease occasionally develop an encephalitis, either prior to (a difficult diagnosis) or concurrent with enlarged lymph nodes. Group A streptococcal infection may lead to peritonsillar abscess, and infectious mononucleosis (Epstein Barr virus) has been associated with both splenic rupture and liver failure. In children with AIDS, cytomegalovirus (CMV) may lead to retinitis.

Further Discussion

Rochalimea (Bartonella) hensleae was convincingly demonstrated to be the cause of cat scratch disease in the mid 1990's in a series of studies from the CDC. The same organism causes bacillary angiomatosis in patients with HIV. The diagnosis of cat scratch disease can now be confirmed by serologic testing. Previously, clinicians relied on skin testing, but the reagents were neither standardized nor approved.

A 3-year-old girl presents to the emergency department refusing to walk. Her mother noted this yesterday evening. There is no history of any trauma. She has been well without any fever or upper respiratory tract symptoms. On physical examination there is no obvious swelling or ecchymosis of the involved extremity. She refuses to put her foot down. Although she cries when you touch her almost anywhere, she seems to be most tender in the lower part of her leg.

1. Which management plan would you follow?
    A. An X-ray of the entire lower extremity
    B. An X-ray from the knee to the foot
    C. A bone scan
    D. An ultrasound of the hip
    E. A hip X-ray

DISCUSSION

ANSWERS:
1. **B. An X-ray from the knee to the foot**

1. Toddlers who limp can challenge the physician's assessment skills. Complete palpation of the abdomen, lower back, pelvis, and lower extremities should be followed by a careful neurologic, skin and foot examination. Occasionally, it is helpful to guide the parent through these maneuvers with the frightened toddler in order to gauge tenderness. Often it is safest to obtain radiographs of the entire lower extremity, but with localized pain, as in this case, one can focus on the suspicious area, at least for the initial study. Thus, the correct answer is to get an X-ray from the knee to the foot.

Further Discussion

Due to several anatomic features, children are more likely than adults to have fractures with low energy injuries. Additionally, they have more subtle physical examination findings associated with the types of fractures that are commonly seen. There are no absolute rules regarding when to obtain X-rays in children who limp; however, you might consider doing so in those who refuse to bear weight, have any focal abnormalities, or show systemic signs or symptoms. This child has the so called "Toddler's" fracture or spiral fracture of the tibia, which is commonly seen in children between the ages of 12 and 36 months. Typically, these appear in the lower third of the tibia, are non- or minimally displaced, and are subtle on plain films of the tibia. In the example provided, a fracture line is apparent but difficult to visualize. If the anteroposterior and lateral X-rays do not reveal any findings and you suspect this type of injury, consider obtaining oblique views. Also, these patients may be evaluated with a bone scan or a second set of films, obtained at 10 to 14 days, looking for periosteal elevation associated with fracture healing. Remember that it is not unusual for such patients to have normal films. Presumptive treatment in the emergency department with splinting and outpatient orthopedic referral is an excellent approach.

When the toddler has the typical radiographic findings and there are no other risk factors revealed during your interview, child abuse is unlikely to be the cause, even if a specific traumatic event cannot be identified.

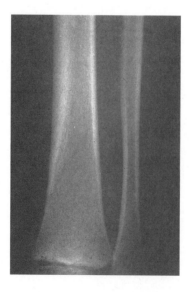

A 3-year-old is brought to the emergency department for a rash. Her mother has noted circular lesions on her skin. These have appeared progressively, first on her buttocks, then on her back, and now on her chest wall. She has no other symptoms. The rash is noted below.

1. Based on the appearance of these lesions you diagnose:
   A. Erythema chronicum migrans
   B. Nummular eczema
   C. Bullous impetigo
   D. Tinea corporis
   E. Discoid lupus

2. Your treatment of the condition is:
   A. Corticosteroids orally
   B. Corticosteroids topically
   C. Diphenhydramine orally
   D. Anti-fungal agents topically
   E. Antibiotics orally

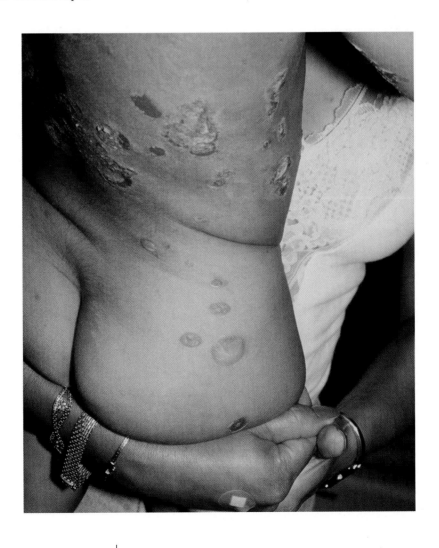

DISCUSSION

ANSWERS:
1. C. **Bullous impetigo**
2. E. **Antibiotics orally**

1. The findings are those of bullous impetigo, which should be treated in this case with oral antibiotics. The most common organism for this infection is *Staphylococcus aureus*. Tinea corporis is also circular, but causes usually just one or two lesions that have a microvesicular margin. Nummular eczema is scaling and occurs in areas of dry skin; other eczematoid skin changes may be apparent. Discoid lupus is rare in children, and in particular, rare at this age. It is a chronic skin condition with systemic manifestations. Erythema chronicum migrans is the hallmark of Lyme disease and consists of a large, erythematous, circular lesion or a series of concentric circles.

2. Although topical antibiotic therapy, with mupirocin, is effective for impetigo, when a number of lesions and numerous sites are involved, children should be treated with oral antibiotics. Logical choices, based on the expected organisms, include erythromycin and cephalexin.

Further Discussion

There are several reasons to treat impetigo adequately and promptly, above and beyond simply making the lesions disappear. Antibiotic therapy reduces the likelihood that the organisms will invade deeper structures and cause cellulitis or adenitis and may also decrease the incidence of acute post-streptococcal glomerulonephritis, which may complicate streptococcal impetigo. Additionally, eradication of the pathogens limits the transmission of this highly contagious infection.

A 6-year-old boy fell from the top of a "monkey bar" and struck a lower bar, before landing on the grass. He had no loss of consciousness and, after the fall, went home. Later in the afternoon, he complained of upper abdominal pain and didn't eat much supper. The following morning, this pain had worsened so his mother brought him to the hospital. On physical examination, he had a pulse of 140/min, a respiratory rate of 38/min, and a temperature of 38.3°C. His heart and lung exam were normal.

1. His most likely diagnosis is:
    A. Laceration of the liver
    B. Duodenal hematoma
    C. Transverse process fracture
    D. Fractured pancreas
    E. Perforated viscus

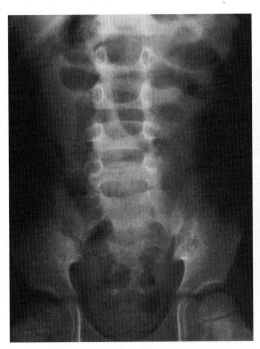
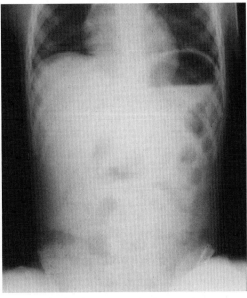

DISCUSSION

ANSWER:

1. **E. Perforated viscus**

1. Pneumoperitoneum following blunt trauma may result from perforation of a hollow viscus. Although pneumoperitoneum is uncommonly seen in children, in addition to being post-traumatic, it can occur as a complication of appendicitis, intestinal ischemia, ulcer disease, inflammatory bowel disease, and ingested foreign bodies. Although the amount of air is usually quite small, plain X-rays are able to detect it in most cases, as demonstrated here. Laceration of the liver or a fractured pancreas might immediately follow the type of blunt injury sustained by this boy, but these lesions would manifest on X-ray with an ileus, rather than free air; CT is needed to make a specific diagnosis. Duodenal hematomas generally cause vomiting 1-2 days after a blow to the abdomen. X-rays may show a proximal small bowel obstruction. Fracture of a transverse process requires a significant force, as is seen in motor vehicle accidents or falls from heights greater than those which occur from playground equipment; these injuries may occur in isolation but should lead one to expect additionally pathology, particularly involving the kidneys.

Further Discussion

In this patient's erect X-rays, air is visualized beneath the right diaphragm leaflet (Figure). The right hemi-diaphragm is seen as a very thin structure, as opposed to left thicker line. The left shadow represents the stomach wall and the diaphragm leaflet together. On the supine film, air can often be seen lying over the liver, as is the case in this example. Outlining of the intestinal wall due to gas present on the serosal and mucosal sides may also be a clue. The cross table lateral or left lateral decubitus technique may be employed in young infants and toddlers in whom the preferred upright X-ray is difficult to obtain. As the evaluating physician, it is important to order appropriate views. The requested series should include a flat plate and upright or decubitus view of the abdomen, in addition to an upright chest film.

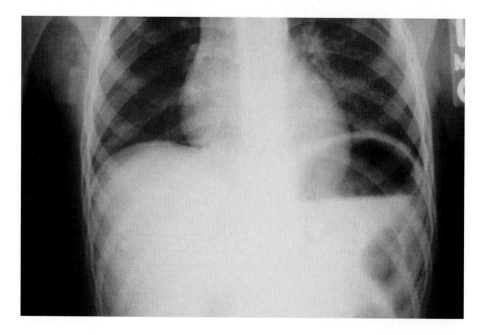

A 4-year-old awoke with swelling of his left eye and fever. After watching his swelling increase during the morning, his parents brought him to the emergency department. There is no history of trauma. His past medical history is negative, and he is fully immunized. His vital signs are P 110/min, R 26/min, BP 110/60 mm Hg, and T 39.5°C. The findings are limited to those shown in the photograph below. The eyelid is warm and tender to palpation.

1. Based on these findings the most likely diagnosis is:
   A. Insect bite
   B. Periorbital cellulitis
   C. Trauma
   D. Maxillary sinusitis
   E. Blepharitis

2. Of the following, which is the most important test to do immediately?
   A. Complete blood count
   B. Culture of the blood
   C. Culture of the conjunctiva
   D. CT scan of the orbit
   E. Fluorescein staining of the cornea

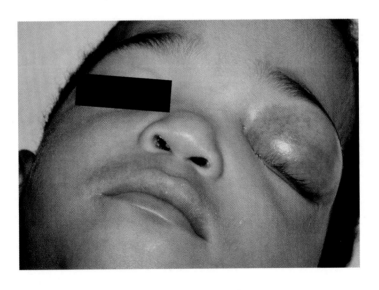

DISCUSSION

ANSWERS:
1. **B. Periorbital cellulitis.**
2. **D. CT scan of the orbit**

1. The diagnosis is periorbital cellulitis. It is helpful to perform a careful physical examination to rule out orbital cellulitis, looking for proptosis and restriction of extraocular movement. Insect bites can cause eyelid swelling to this degree, but there are usually bites scattered over the surface of the body, a history of itching, and no fever. Trauma should always be considered, even in the absence of a specific history for injury; it does not cause fever and would be unlikely to be confined to just the upper eyelid. Maxillary sinusitis might cause lymphedema or extend directly into the soft tissues, but one would expect lower lid and malar swelling first, followed by upper lid swelling. It is important to look for sinusitis underlying periorbital cellulitis, as it may indicate the need for a longer course of antibiotic therapy. Blepharitis or conjunctivitis leads to eyelid swelling, but there is always a history of crusting of the eyes at the onset of the processes. When the caked and matted lids are treated roughly, swelling ensues.

2. The most important test to order is a CT scan of the orbit, to exclude orbital cellulitis. With this degree of swelling, it may be difficult to distinguish orbital from periorbital infection, as physical examination is limited by pain and edema. Orbital cellulitis may cause a fluctuant collection and require immediate surgical drainage to relieve pressure on the optic nerve. Periorbital cellulitis is treated with antibiotics, which should be administered intravenously with extensive local disease, as seen here, or when a bacteremic infection is suspected.

Further Discussion

Periorbital cellulitis used to be caused predominantly by *Hemophilus influenzae*. With the widespread use of Hib vaccine, *H. influenzae* is no longer the predominant organism. In this case, group A beta hemolytic *Streptococcus* was the offending microbial agent. *Streptococcus pneumoniae* and *Staphylococcus aureus* are other potential pathogens.

A father brings his 2-year-old son to the emergency department because he has been unwilling or unable to walk. Yesterday he fell over his tricycle while playing inside on a carpeted floor. Since then, he has refused to walk or crawl. He has otherwise been well without fever or upper respiratory tract illness. He is on no medications and has no chronic health problems. His general physical examination is normal. You have difficulty locating any discrete area of focal tenderness, and there is no swelling or ecchymosis noted. Despite enticing him with interesting toys and delicious cherry popsicles from across the room, you are unable to get him to use his injured extremity.

1. You recommend the following
   A. Follow up in 2-3 days
   B. Aspiration of the knee joint
   C. A long leg cast
   D. Operative intervention
   E. Intravenous antibiotics

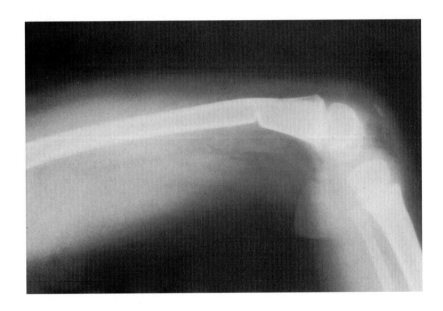

DISCUSSION

ANSWERS:

1. C. A long leg cast

1. It is concerning that this child refuses to bear weight; thus, an evaluation including radiographs is appropriate. This boy has a torus or buckle fracture, which is consistent with the minor mechanism of injury described by the father. On the radiograph, you see slight bending of the distal femur with buckling of the periosteum on one side. Always carefully follow the periosteum as many fractures are much more subtle than this one. Casting alleviates pain, protects from secondary injury and promotes healing. Neither closed nor open manipulation is necessary. Extremity shortening and angulation are rarely problems for children with these fractures. If one noted periosteal elevation, suggesting osteomyelitis, intravenous antibiotics would be a consideration. With septic arthritis of the knee, X-rays may show an effusion in the joint space; aspiration confirms the diagnosis and provides a specimen for culture. The most common reason for limp in an afebrile child is toxic synovitis, which causes no radiographic abnormalities. These patients need only a brief course of anti-inflammatory therapy and follow-up to make sure that an early infection has not been missed.

Further Discussion

The anatomy of children's bones differs from that of adolescents and adults and predisposes them to different types of injuries. First, the bone of growing children is more porous with an extensive, parallel Haversian canal system making it susceptible to bowing or plastic bending, torus or buckle, and greenstick fractures. Second, ligaments are the strongest component of the skeleton, followed by bones and finally the growth plates. Thus, growth plate injuries and fractures are more common than sprains. Finally, the periosteum is thick and strong promoting rapid healing, extensive remodeling, and decreased movement of fracture fragments during injury. Physical findings may be very subtle. It has been suggested in the adult population that the presence of deformity, swelling, and ecchymosis correlate with fracture. If this approach were to be used in children, many fractures would be missed on the first visit.

A previously healthy, 6-year-old boy comes to the emergency department after experiencing his first seizure. He has had an upper respiratory infection for several days along with a low grade fever. His mother has been treating him with pseudoephedrine.

Vital signs:	P 75/min R 22/min BP 92/56 mm Hg T 38.2°C
General	Mildly lethargic
Eyes	No conjunctivitis
Ears	Tympanic membranes pearly gray
Nodes	No adenopathy
Neck	Supple
Lungs	No rales or wheezes
Heart	No murmurs
Abdomen	No tenderness
Neurologic	No focal findings

1. After securing intravenous access, your next step is:
   A. Adenosine intravenously
   B. Ceftriaxone intravenously
   C. Cardiology consultation
   D. Head CT scan
   E. Fosphenytoin intravenously

2. With further questioning, you learn that the boy has a history of:
   A. Retinitis pigmentosa
   B. Kawasaki disease
   C. Myocarditis
   D. Atrial septal defect
   E. Sensorineural deafness

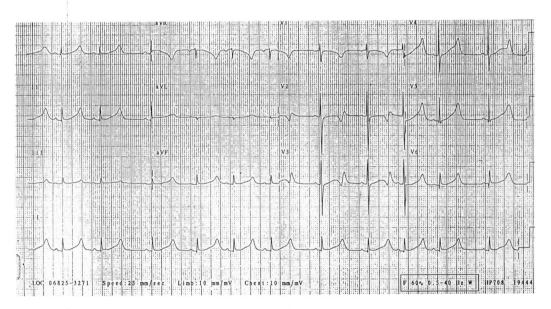

(EKG courtesy of Mary Chris Burley, M.D.)

DISCUSSION

ANSWERS:

1. C. Cardiology consultation
2. E. Sensorineural deafness

1. The EKG shows a prolonged QT interval. Since patients with prolonged QT syndrome are at risk for sudden death, it would be appropriate to consult a cardiologist about therapy before discharge from the emergency department. The EKG does not show supraventricular tachycardia, so adenosine is not indicated. While either ceftriaxone for possible meningitis or a head CT scan to look for a mass lesion might be reasonable in evaluating some seizures, neither would represent a next step, given the finding of the abnormal QT interval.

2. A prolonged QT interval may be an isolated finding or occur in association with several syndromes. One such syndrome includes sensorineural deafness as a component. None of the conditions listed that involve (myocarditis, atrial septal defect), or potentially affect (Kawasaki Disease) the heart, cause prolongation of the QT interval.

Further Discussion

Prolonged QT syndrome may manifest at any point during childhood or remain occult until later in life. Common presentations include syncope, seizures, and sudden death. Because of the association with seizures, I generally recommend an EKG on every patient with a first afebrile convulsion (but not those with simple febrile seizures). The normal values for the QT interval vary with the rate of the heart, and thus with age as well. After measuring the interval (from the start of the QRS complex to the end of the T wave), one must either consult a standard table of normal values or correct for heart rate. The later is accomplished by dividing the square root of the RR interval into the measured QT interval. The resulting value should be less than 0.45.

A 3-week-old boy arrives in the emergency department with a 1-day history of lethargy and vomiting. He was a full term infant, born vaginally after a normal pregnancy to a healthy young mother. He is breastfed and has had some problems with "spitting" since birth, although his weight gain has been adequate. His last episodes of vomiting appeared greenish to his mother, so she brought him to the hospital. On physical examination, his vital signs are as follows: P 180/min, R 53/min, BP 58/32 mm Hg, and T 36° C. He is lethargic and pale, with a flat fontanelle. Breath sounds are clear, but he grunts occasionally. His extremities are mottled. His abdomen is distended and firm to palpation.

1. This most likely diagnosis is:
    A. Pyloric stenosis
    B. Duodenal atresia
    C. Inguinal hernia
    D. Sepsis
    E. Malrotation

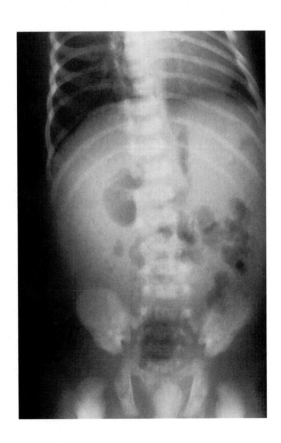

DISCUSSION

ANSWERS:

1. E. Malrotation

1. Bilious vomiting in the neonate is presumed to be due to obstruction. In a neonate presenting with such symptoms, a catastrophic abdominal emergency should be suspected. This infant has malrotation. Pyloric stenosis often presents at this age but does not cause bilious vomiting, while duodenal atresia causes bilious vomiting but manifests within the first 2 days of life. When present, an incarcerated inguinal hernia is obvious on physical examination; distal small bowel obstruction may ensue. A septic infant may have bilious vomiting and an ileus, but not frank obstruction.

Further Discussion

Malrotation results from failure of normal rotation of the midgut leading to abnormal fixation of the mesentery. Normally the mesentery extends from the left upper quadrant to the right lower quadrant, with the duodeno-jejunal junction to the left of the ligament of Treitz and the superior mesenteric artery. This long mesenteric attachment prevents twisting. In the case of malrotation, the mesenteric attachment is short, allowing for twisting around the superior mesenteric artery. Obstruction also results from bands of peritoneum crossing anterior to the bowel, most commonly at the third portion of the duodenum.

The majority of patients present in the neonatal period with bilious vomiting, abdominal distension and pain. In older patients, the diagnosis is more challenging. They may present with a history of feeding problems and formula intolerance with vomiting, or with poor growth. Abdominal radiograph findings are variable. As with many other disease processes, the plain films may be remarkably normal. There may be evidence of proximal obstruction with a dilated stomach, or a "double-bubble" sign with a paucity of gas distally. An upper gastrointestinal study is the study of choice to make the diagnosis. As in this example, the duodenal loop may appear dilated with obstruction at the third portion.

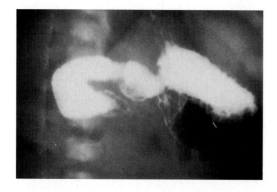

A 2-month-old infant is brought to the emergency department for a rash of the buttocks. The parents state that the rash appeared 15 minutes after the infant, wearing his diaper, had spent about 10 minutes in the freshly chlorinated pool at a neighbor's house. They deny any recent illness or prior dermatologic conditions.

1. This rash most likely represents:
    A. Candidiasis
    B. Staphylococcal infection
    C. Chemical irritation
    D. Scald burn
    E. Physical trauma

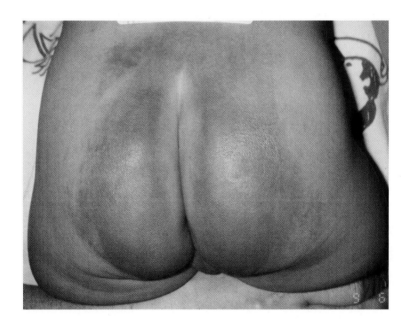

DISCUSSION

ANSWERS:

1. **C. Chemical irritation**

1. This rash is the result of a chemical burn due to a high concentration of chlorine (in an improperly treated pool), which was absorbed by the lining of the diaper, resulting in a prolonged exposure over the buttocks. While one might rightfully question this explanation initially, the findings do not support either a scald burn or mechanical trauma. A scald burn would have involved the intergluteal crease, and erythema from slapping would not likely be absolutely symmetric and confined precisely to the diaper area. Candidiasis does not have an abrupt onset, is usually most intense in the creases, and often includes satellite lesions. Staphylococcal infections in the diaper area manifest as either impetigo or pustulosis.

Further Discussion

Although chemical burns are rare, diaper rash is common. The usual causes include irritation to the skin and candidiasis. At times, more generalized dermatologic disorders, such as atopic dermatitis or seborrhea, may manifest initially in the perineal region. Bacterial infections are seen occasionally.

A 13-year-old boy fell onto his outstretched hands while playing ice hockey. He comes to the emergency department with a swollen hand. He has no other injuries or complaints.

1. A complication of this injury is:
   A. Avascular necrosis of the distal fragment
   B. Avascular necrosis of the proximal fragment
   C. Osteoarthritis of the wrist
   D. Radial nerve neuropathy
   E. None of the above

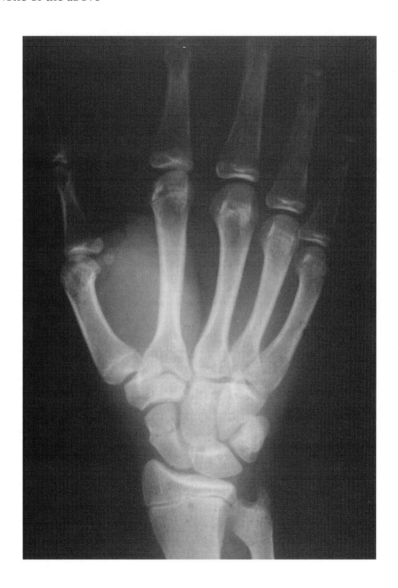

DISCUSSION

ANSWER:

1. **B. Avascular necrosis of the proximal fragment**

1. This is an example of a scaphoid or navicular fracture. The proximal fracture fragment is at risk for avascular necrosis if the blood supply is damaged, and the risk of non-union is not insignificant. In the pediatric patient, the distal third of the scaphoid is commonly involved in the fracture, and complications of non-union and avascular necrosis are rare.

Further Discussion

In general, fractures around the wrist of pediatric patients usually involve the growth plate. Carpal bone fractures are exceedingly rare as these bones are protected by thick cartilage. Occasionally, you will see such a fracture in the adolescent patient.

A fall on an outstretched arm in conjunction with wrist hyperextension is the usual mechanism of injury. Most patients will have soft tissue swelling along with tenderness in the anatomic "snuff box."

The radiograph findings may be subtle or absent initially, emphasizing the importance of the clinical diagnosis. Oblique radiographs enhance the ability to visualize the fracture line. In this example, however, a fracture line is readily seen. Radiographic findings include soft tissue swelling, the presence of a fracture line or an irregular cortical border, shortening of the bone and increased density of one of the fracture fragments due to rotation. In the adult, the fracture usually occurs at the waist of the scaphoid bone.

Patients with this injury require casting from below the elbow to the metacarpal heads and the interphalangeal joint of the thumb for a period of 4 to 6 weeks. For patients with pain at the snuff box but normal radiographs, splinting and orthopedic follow-up are appropriate. X-rays taken at a later date often reveal the presence of a healing fracture.

An 8-year-old boy lacerated his forearm when he accidentally put it through the window of a storm door.

1. The structure that is most likely to have been injured is the:
    A. Radial artery
    B. Flexor carpi ulnaris tendon
    C. Median nerve
    D. Palmaris longus tendon
    E. Flexor digitorum superficialis tendon

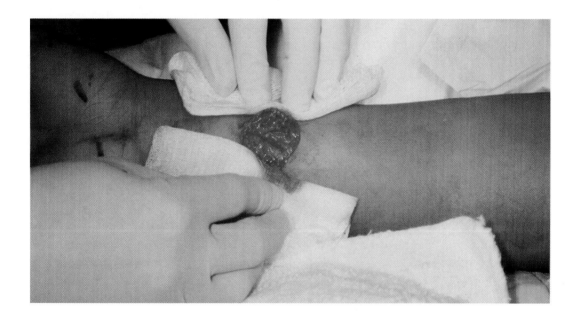

DISCUSSION

ANSWER:

1. D. Palmaris longus tendon

1. The palmaris longus is the most superficial tendon in the forearm and is located centrally, making it vulnerable with lacerations in this region. Of the structures listed, only the median nerve is located in the area of this wound, though deep to the palmaris longus. The flexor carpi ulnaris is deeper and more toward the ulnar aspect of the forearm, while the radial artery and the flexor digitorum superficialis are deeper (despite the name of the latter) and on the radial aspect.

Further Discussion

In this particular case, the tendon is exposed but not injured. Although the palmaris longus has no essential functions, one needs to be certain not to confuse it with any of its neighbors, particularly the flexor carpi radialis. Remember that laceration of the palmaris longus serves as a reminder to carefully explore the wound and perform an appropriate neurovascular evaluation, as these injuries indicate that the penetration of the forearm has extended beyond the superficial layers. Of particular importance, flexor tendons that are completely lacerated may retract such that the injury is not readily apparent.

A 2-year-old is transported from another hospital for further treatment of wheezing. Her therapy there consisted of albuterol nebulizations, supplemental oxygen, and intravenous steroids. She remains tachypneic with moderate work of breathing. She has had no previous episodes of wheezing, and except for some clear rhinorrhea, she has been well. After arrival at your emergency department, you find that she is wheezing on the left side only.

1. Which of the following would you do next:
   A. Obtain a lateral neck X-ray
   B. Start intravenous terbutaline
   C. Place a chest tube
   D. Consult otolaryngology
   E. Perform indirect laryngoscopy

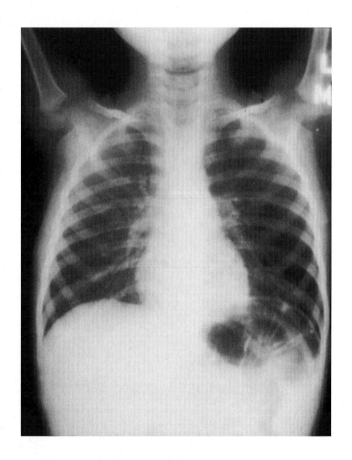

DISCUSSION

ANSWER:

1. **D. Consult otolaryngology**

1. The differential diagnosis of the wheezing patient, especially during the toddler years, includes the possibility of a foreign body. This child has no previous history of bronchospasm and is at the perfect age for foreign body aspiration. Thus, the finding of a lucent area in one lung strongly suggests the need for rigid bronchoscopy by otolaryngology in the operating suite, rather than flexible laryngoscopy in the emergency department. Since there is no pneumothorax, a chest tube is not indicated. Although intravenous terbutaline is effective in severe asthma, it will not relieve bronchospasm from a foreign body. Finally, a lateral neck X-ray offers no additional information, as the problem has been localized to the lung.

Further Discussion

With foreign body aspiration, the symptoms produced and the radiographic findings are dependent upon the location of the foreign body and whether or not any obstruction is complete or incomplete. At the laryngeal level, the child may have a hoarse voice or refuse to talk. Foreign bodies causing incomplete obstruction in the trachea or bronchi may result in tachypnea, wheezing, and diminished breath sounds, although the physical examination may be remarkably normal.

This patient has air trapping on the left side on the chest radiograph. When evaluating a chest radiograph, differential aeration is an important finding . During inspiration, the airway dilates and air passes beyond the foreign body. During exhalation, the airway naturally narrows and air is trapped in the airways and lung tissue distal to the foreign body. The involved lung or portion of the lung will look blacker than the normal lung due to air trapping as well as decreased blood flow. This finding is accentuated with inspiration and expiration. Practically speaking, obtaining inspiratory and expiratory views is nearly impossible with babies and toddlers. Physicians caring for children often substitute lateral decubitus X-rays in an attempt to document this differential aeration. In the decubitus position, the dependent lung normally empties more and the mediastinum falls to that side. The absence of this finding suggests the presence of air trapping. In the presence of complete bronchial obstruction, the distal portion of the lung becomes atelectatic. In the example provided, note that the left lung does not empty as well as the right lung when the patient is in the left decubitus position.

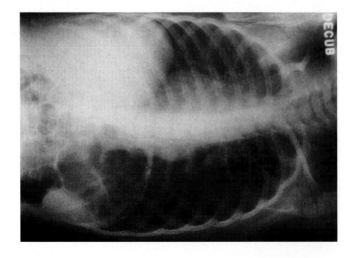

A 2-year-old patient has had a fever for 24 hours and the parents report that the child is sleeping more than usual. On examination, you observe lethargy, a fever of 39.8°C, and mild nuchal rigidity. There are no focal neurologic findings.

1. When performing a lumbar puncture as shown, you would use a:
   A. 22 gauge, 1.5 inch needle
   B. 22 gauge, 2.5 inch needle
   C. 20 gauge, 2.5 inch needle
   D. 20 gauge, 3.5 inch needle
   E. 18 gauge, 1.5 inch needle

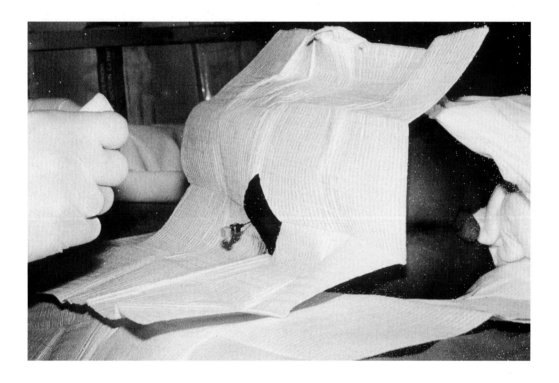

DISCUSSION

ANSWER:

1. **B. 22 gauge, 1.5 inch needle**

1. For a 2-year-old child, a 22 gauge 1.5 inch needle is most appropriate. Shorter needles are easier to control when attempting a lumbar puncture on a squirming child, and thereby reduce the likelihood of a traumatic tap. Thus, I would prefer a 1.5 inch needle over a 2.5 inch needle for this patient, although the latter is acceptable. A larger gauge is unnecessary and will only create a greater chance of a persistent cerebrospinal fluid (CSF) leak.

Further Discussion

Two other issues that arise around lumbar puncture are the use of local anesthetic agents and sedatives. In terms of the former, one can make an argument for using local anesthesia at all ages, since it has been well demonstrated that infants perceive pain and react to it physiologically. Others would claim that in a small baby, the injection of lidocaine obscures the landmarks, making multiple attempts and traumatic punctures more likely, and that it causes as much pain as a single pass with a 22 gauge spinal needle. Certainly, beyond the first 6 months, I strongly recommend local anesthesia, if for no other reason than for facilitation of the actual procedure, by decreasing movement of the patients on initial contact between the skin and the spinal needle. Sedation should be used when indicated. I rarely sedate a child under age 3 years or over 12 years for a lumbar puncture, relying instead on appropriate local anesthesia.

A previously healthy 11-year-old boy comes to the emergency department with a history of palpitations on and off over 5 days. Over the past year, he has had several similar episodes, usually limited to 1-2 days. One week prior to the visit, his father reports that he fell approximately 15 feet from a tree branch onto his chest but seemed to require no medical attention at that time. He has been using an oral decongestant for the past few days to treat a mild upper respiratory infection. His vital signs are as follows: P 76/min, R 18/min, BP 110/70 mm Hg, and T 37.4°C. The remainder of the physical examination is normal except for a grade I/VI systolic ejection murmur, best heard along the left sternal border.

1. This child's problem is:
    A. Congenital
    B. Traumatic
    C. Infectious
    D. Toxicologic
    E. Emotional

2. You recommend:
    A. Echocardiography
    B. Oral flecainide
    C. Observation in the ICU
    D. Intravenous adenosine
    E. No further measures

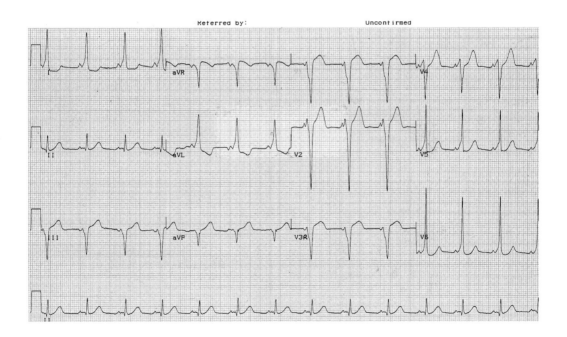

DISCUSSION

ANSWERS:
1. A. Congenital
2. B. Oral flecainide

1. This boy has Wolff-Parkinson-White syndrome (WPW), which is a congenital conduction anomaly due to the presence of a bypass tract. His EKG shows a short PR interval, a wide QRS complex, and a slurred upstroke to the QRS that is most notable in leads I, V5, and V6. There is the appearance of left axis deviation, left ventricular hypertrophy, and ST-T wave abnormalities, which actually reflect the conduction disturbance. Patients with WPW are prone to develop supraventricular tachycardia (SVT), explaining this patient's palpitations. Trauma may cause a myocardial contusion, which may be accompanied by ST segment elevation or, more often, a completely normal EKG. Contusions of the heart in children are uncommon, generally occur only after a severe impact, and usually manifest within the first 24-48 hours after injury. The use of sympathomimetic agents in decongestants has been associated with the development of SVT, but the EKG is normal between episodes of tachycardia. Myocarditis may follow a minor respiratory infection but does not lead to SVT or the electrocardiographic findings on this tracing. Although anxiety is by far the most frequent etiology for palpitation in adolescents, as always this diagnosis is one of exclusion.

2. Flecainide, which slows conduction through both the AV node and the bypass tract, is a reasonable therapeutic option for a child with episodes of SVT from WPW. Although adenosine is the drug of choice for SVT, it is used to "break" an episode of tachycardia rather than for prophylaxis, as its half life is 10-20 seconds. Echocardiography would be a useful adjunct to evaluate myocardial function in patients suspected of either myocarditis or cardiac contusion; both of these diagnoses generally merit observation in an ICU. Although some patients with WPW require no therapy, given the frequency of episodes in this patient, observation at home would not be an optimal strategy.

Further Discussion

Generally, the decision to initiate therapy with any anti-arrhythmic drug in a child with WPW syndrome would be made only after consultation with a pediatric cardiologist. Long-term monitoring or electrophysiologic studies are needed in many cases to elucidate the extent and severity of the problem. Options include observation, pharmacotherapy, and radiofrequency or surgical ablation of the bypass tract.

A 12-month-old girl comes to the emergency department in the early evening with a 1-day history of intermittent irritability and crying. Her parents describe periods of inconsolability, lasting 5-15 minutes, and a single episode of vomiting. The girl ate cereal in the morning but was not interested in her bottle since then. For the past week, she and her siblings have had "colds." Over the course of the afternoon, she became more sleepy and her mother's concern mounted. Her physical examination reveals a listless 12-month-old with the following vital signs: P 150/min, R 24/min, BP 100/60 mm Hg, and T 37.8°C. Her tympanic membranes are clear. No abnormal lung sounds or cardiac murmurs are appreciated. The abdomen in not distended or tender, but the bowel sounds are decreased. There is full range of motion of all joints.

1. Given this clinical scenario, her most likely diagnosis is:
   A. Meningitis
   B. Gastroenteritis
   C. Appendicitis
   D. Pneumonia
   E. Intussusception

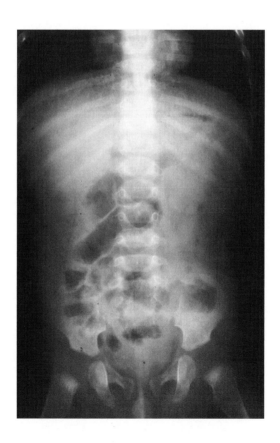

DISCUSSION

ANSWERS:

1. E. Intussusception

1. This child most likely has intussusception, given both the clinical findings and the presence of a "sentinel loop" of distended bowel. Although gastroenteritis is a possible explanation, I would consider it a diagnosis of exclusion in this case, since the child has had episodic irritability without either fever or diarrhea and the abdominal X-ray is concerning. Appendicitis is unusual in the first two years of life, and often presents only after perforation with high fever and signs of sepsis and abdominal tenderness, when the age of the patient allows detection of this finding. Pneumonia doesn't cause episodic irritability and is not seen in the lower lobes on the X-ray. Certainly, meningitis is a cause of irritability; however, the irritability either increases or changes to lethargy. Additionally, meningitis (especially bacterial) without fever is distinctly unusual outside the neonatal period.

Further Discussion

Intussusception is typically seen in children between the ages of 6 months and 2 years. It is caused by invagination of one portion of the intestine into another.

The findings on plain radiographs of the abdomen are variable and, to a certain extent, dependent upon the duration of the symptoms and the location of the intussusception. Early on, abdominal X-rays are usually completely normal. A paucity of gas in the right lower quadrant, resulting in poor definition of the liver edge, may be seen. As time progresses, findings consistent with small bowel obstruction may ensue. Rarely, an edematous intussusceptum may be visible, outlined by air within the bowel. Eventually, a perforation may develop, with the radiographic finding of free air in the abdomen. This patient's X-rays reveal the so-called "sentinel loop" which is a localized ileus occurring in a portion of bowel lying next to an inflamed organ. With the introduction of barium (figure below), the site of obstruction is identified.

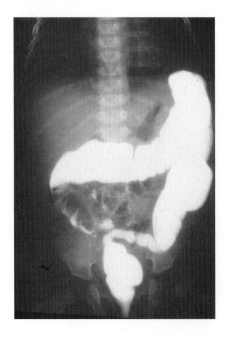

The parents of a 7-year-old boy report that he has been drinking excessive amounts of fluids and urinating large volumes for 10 days. They feel that he has lost at least 5 pounds of weight during this time. On examination, his vital signs are as follows: P 184/min, R 32/min, and BP 82/40 mm Hg. He appears acutely ill and his mucous membranes are dry. To achieve venous access, you cannulate a vessel in his neck.

1. Your success is facilitated by the use of a "J" wire because:
    A. The dome of the lung rises above the level of the clavicle on the right
    B. The carotid artery lies medial to the internal jugular vein at this point
    C. The external jugular vein joins the subclavian vein at an acute angle
    D. A straight wire may perforate the junction of the subclavian and jugular veins
    E. A "J" wire is less likely than a straight wire to lead to cardiac tamponade

2. The most common complication of this procedure is:
    A. Arterial cannulation
    B. Hemothorax
    C. Pneumothorax
    D. Hematoma
    E. Cerebrovascular accident

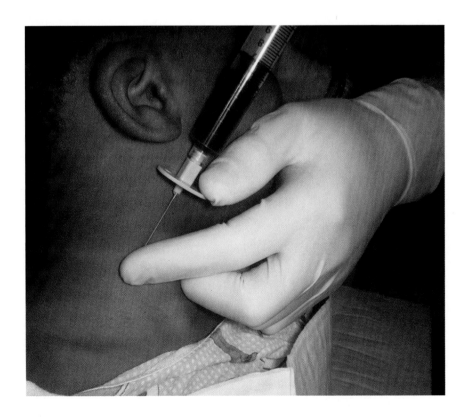

DISCUSSION

ANSWERS:

1. C. The external jugular vein joins the subclavian vein at an acute angle
2. D. Hematoma

1. The physician is catheterizing the external jugular vein, as indicated by the location and orientation of the needle. The external jugular vein courses across the mid portion of the sternocleidomastoid muscle, from medial to lateral, as it descends. Use of a "J" wire facilitates cannulation of the central circulation via the external jugular vein because the external jugular and subclavian veins join at an acute angle, which may be difficult to negotiate with a straight wire, particularly in children under 3 years old. The rise of the right lung dome above the clavicle and the position of the carotid artery are relevant to catheterization of the internal, rather than the external, jugular vein. Any type of wire or catheter may cause a perforation (potentially leading to tamponade if the right atrium is involved), but this event is not more likely with either type of wire.

2. Cannulation of the external jugular vein rarely leads to complications other than a hematoma in the neck, which has no consequences, except occasionally in patients with a severe bleeding diathesis. Both pneumothorax and hemothorax are remote possibilities. Inadvertent cannulation of the carotid artery may occur when attempting to access the internal jugular vein. The external jugular vein bears no direct relationship to the intracranial circulation, and cannulation is not complicated by cerebrovascular accidents.

CASE 110

A 4-year-old girl is referred for evaluation of persistent fever and new onset torticollis. She saw her pediatrician 8 days ago and was diagnosed with pharyngitis and otitis media, for which she received a course of amoxicillin. There was initial improvement, but over the past several days the fever and sore throat have returned. During the past 24 hours, she has held her head cocked to one side and has refused to eat or drink. The family members deny the possibility of an accidental ingestion. On physical examination, her temperature is 39.5°C, her respiratory rate is 28/min, and she is mildly ill-appearing with torticollis. There is no nystagmus, and her throat appears normal. She is neurologically intact. The WBC is 26,000/mm^3 with 5% bands and 80% neutrophils.

1. The girl needs which treatment?
    A. Endotracheal intubation in the OR
    B. Racemic epinephrine in the ICU
    C. Endoscopy in the emergency department
    D. Antibiotics in the hospital
    E. I & D in the emergency department

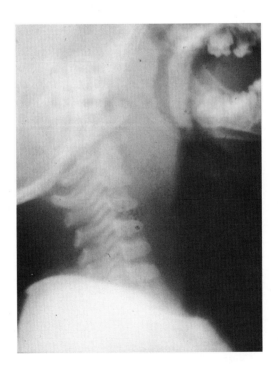

DISCUSSION

ANSWERS:

1. **D. Antibiotics in the hospital**

1. This child has a retropharyngeal abscess, a bacterial infection in the lymphoid tissue in the potential space lying between the esophagus and the cervical vertebrae. Some cases respond to intravenous antibiotic alone, while others require incision and drainage in the operating room (unlike peritonsillar abscesses which are usually drained in the emergency department). Patients with epiglottitis are managed with endotracheal intubation in the operating room when time allows; these radiographs show a normal, rather than a swollen, epiglottis. Severe croup, which often causes laryngeal edema seen on X-ray, may respond to nebulized racemic epinephrine (as well as other beta adrenergic agents) given in the emergency department, a hospital ward, or the ICU. Foreign bodies of the airway are best removed by endoscopy in the operating room in most instances.

Further Discussion

Typically, patients with retropharyngeal infections appear toxic and have fever, sore throat, drooling, stridor and respiratory distress. However, the clinical picture may be altered by pretreatment with oral antibiotics, as in this child.

The retropharyngeal space is notoriously difficult to interpret in the pediatric patient. It is affected by the position of the patient's head and neck and by the phase of inspiration. As seen in this example (see figures below), flexion and inspiration tend to exaggerate the size of the retropharyngeal space, mimicking abscess/cellulitis. In pediatrics, measurement of the soft tissue width is less reliable than in adults. Although the rules state that the prevertebral space should be no wider than half the adjacent vertebral body along the upper half of the cervical spine, the degree of ossification and minor changes in position may influence this relationship.

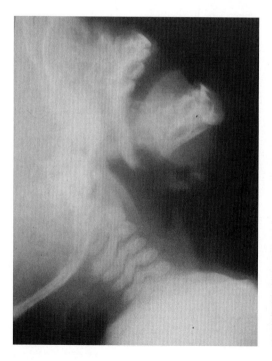 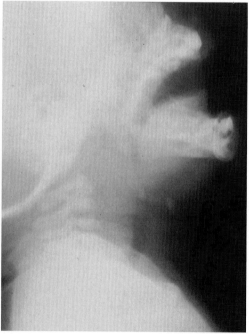

A 6-year-old boy is brought to the emergency department with swelling of his right ear. This was noted by his father when the boy came home from playing after school. The child has a past medical history of frequent ear infections. His father denies recent trauma to the area. The vital signs are: P 100/min, R 20/min, BP 100/68 mm Hg, and T 37°C. The child is well-appearing, except as noted. The ear is warm to the touch, but not tender.

1. The most likely diagnosis is:
   A. Trauma
   B. Mumps
   C. Mastoiditis
   D. Otitis externa
   E. Insect bite

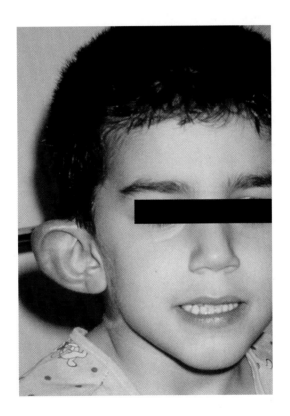

DISCUSSION

ANSWER:

1. **E. Insect bite**

1. An allergic reaction is the most common cause of an acutely swollen, nontender ear, and a local insect bite is the usual precipitant. Occult trauma is always possible in pediatric patients either because they were injured by an adult (parent or teacher) and are afraid of disclosing or because they were injured at play or by another child who may also threaten them not to tell. Children pulled by the ear may have a very similar appearance. A "boxed" ear usually has an ecchymosis on the inner aspect of the pinna. Both mumps and mastoiditis could push the ear into this position, but they would not cause swelling or erythema of the pinna itself. Additionally, mastoiditis should be marked by fever, evidence of otitis media, and tenderness/erythema over the mastoid area. With mumps, one would expect fever and visible swelling of the parotid gland. Otitis externa, or swimmers' ear, produces extreme pain and sometimes purulent discharge. It can spread as a cellulitis into surrounding soft tissues but usually extends anteriorly into the preauricular area, not into the pinna

Further Discussion

Allergic edema is frequently quite pronounced in children when the reaction involves the ear, the eyelid, the lips, or the penis, where loose skin may become quite distended by the accumulation of fluid in the subcutaneous tissues. Particularly during the summer months, these reactions are frequent and are most often from an insect bite. When a local site of entry is not readily apparent or is obscured by edema, a careful search of other regions of the body may reveal typical lesions.

Local allergic reactions of the ears cause swelling, warmth, and some deformity of the pinna, but no pain. The ear may or may not be itchy. Systemic insults are more likely to produce bilateral swelling. Possible treatments for this child are cool compresses and oral diphenhydramine to reduce the swelling.

A 3-year-old arrives with EMTs who were called to the home by his parents when they were unable to arouse him in the morning. On arrival to the emergency department, he is obtunded, hypotensive, and breathing shallowly. You have intubated his trachea and achieved intravenous access.

1. At this point, the most likely diagnosis is:
   A. Hemolytic uremic syndrome
   B. Henoch Schönlein purpura
   C. Acute lymphoblastic leukemia
   D. Meningococcal sepsis
   E. Fulminant hepatitis

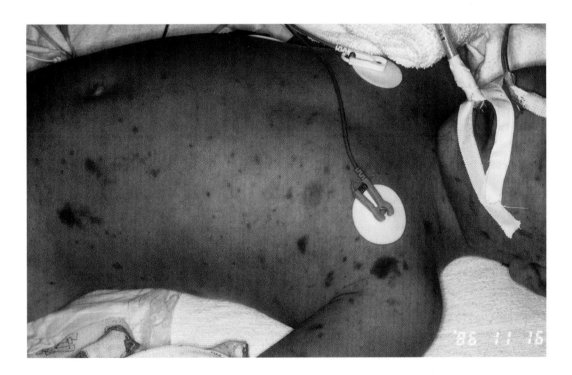

DISCUSSION

ANSWER:

1. **D. Meningococcal sepsis**

1. This youngster has meningococcemia. Frequently, a child with this disease goes to bed with nothing more than a mild, or even unnoticed, fever, only to awaken with overwhelming sepsis. Although hemolytic uremic syndrome (HUS) may cause a purpuric eruption, it usually comes on gradually after a prodromal gastrointestinal illness, which becomes complicated by bloody diarrhea. Rarely do patients with HUS present in profound shock. Henoch Schönlein purpura (HSP) produces a purpuric eruption, often confined to the lower extremities, but is not accompanied by hypotension or systemic toxicity. A child with newly diagnosed acute lymphoblastic leukemia (ALL) will often be both septic and thrombocytopenic. This boy falls in the right age range, but ALL presents less commonly than does meningococcemia with this type of abrupt onset of hemodynamic instability and purpura fulminans. Finally, a bleeding diathesis is a hallmark of fulminant hepatitis, but generally follows a prodromal illness and is usually accompanied by jaundice.

Further Discussion

This child has a life-threatening illness. Given the presentation, he has a substantial risk of mortality or loss of some of his extremities due to purpura fulminans. His disease calls for aggressive monitoring and management, including prompt antibiotic administration (ceftriaxone or cefotaxime), secure venous access (centrally, if needed), arterial catheterization, fluid resuscitation, and institution of "pressors" if the blood pressure does not respond to volume expansion in the first 10-15 minutes, which is almost certainly going to be the case. One needs to be careful to avoid falling into the trap of treating with penicillin alone for meningococcemia, because at the time of presentation, the clinical diagnosis must be septic shock which requires broad spectrum coverage for a variety of potential pathogens. Another potential mistake is to perform a lumbar puncture before starting antibiotics if the procedure is going to delay therapy or compromise the child's status. This boy probably does not have meningeal infection, which occurs uncommonly when the onset of disease is abrupt. Even if he does, the antibiotics you give to treat sepsis are sufficient for the initial therapy of meningitis.

A 3-year-old girl with sickle cell disease comes to the emergency department with her grandmother with a complaint of abdominal pain. While exploring the history, you discover that the girl has seen her physician for this problem three times in the past month or so and that this is the second visit to the emergency department. Her appetite has been decreased and she has lost about 2 pounds over the past month. There has been no change in her bowel habits, although her physician recommended a stool softener. Her grandmother staunchly refuses to take her home until you take care of this problem. The physical examination is normal other than abdominal distension and fullness in the left upper quadrant. You decide to start your investigation by obtaining an abdominal radiograph.

1. You suspect the following:
    A. Constipation
    B. Functional pain
    C. Wilms tumor
    D. Bezoar
    E. Splenomegaly

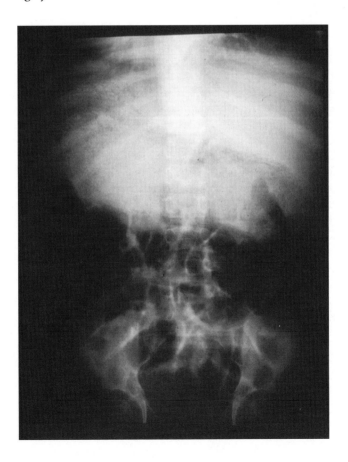

DISCUSSION

ANSWER:

1. D. Bezoar

1. This is an example of a trichobezoar, which accounts for the abdominal pain, the fullness appreciated in the left upper quadrant on physical examination, and the radiographic findings. Functional abdominal pain is the most common cause of abdominal pain in childhood, but it is characterized by a normal examination and a negative X-ray. In the emergency department, this assessment must be a diagnosis of exclusion, as the onus on the physician must always be to rule out emergent conditions, such as appendicitis. Perhaps the second most common reason for abdominal pain in childhood is constipation, which may cause abdominal fullness or the sensation of a mass on palpation (usually in the lower abdomen). Radiographically, abundant stool is visible on the plain X-ray. Although Wilms tumor usually presents in patients at this age and in this fashion (as an asymptomatic abdominal mass), it would not have this radiographic appearance. The spleens of children with sickle cell anemia (hemoglobin SS) autoinfarct by the age of three years. However, splenomegaly does occur in sickle cell anemia during a sequestration crisis or in some of the variants of the disease (e.g., hemoglobin SC disease). With sequestration crisis, the onset is abrupt and the patients appear acutely ill. Once again, the radiographic picture would differ.

Further Discussion

On further questioning of the grandmother once the X-ray had been reviewed, she expressed the concern that her granddaughter ate the hair from the many Barbie dolls in her collection, suggesting the diagnosis of a bezoar. Bezoars arise from ingested indigestible organic matter that forms radio-opaque foreign bodies, most commonly in the stomach. They usually have a granular or foamy appearance and often take the shape of the stomach. The two most common types are trichobezoars (hair) and phytobezoars (vegetable material); other types include lactobezoars (milk; occasionally seen in premature infants) and antacid bezoars. Recently ingested food can mimic a bezoar radiographically, but disappears on subsequent films.

Trichobezoars are most commonly seen in girls in the second decade of life. Occasionally these adolescents have emotional or psychiatric problems. Presenting symptoms include vague abdominal pain, anorexia, weight loss, vomiting, and/or gastric outlet obstruction. It is not unusual to palpate an abdominal mass. Operative removal is usually necessary, at which time the surgeon inspects the bowel for hair balls, a condition given the name the "Rapunzel Syndrome."

A 16-year-old seeks care for a diffuse rash on his torso. He is sexually active and is concerned that this rash may come from his sexual contacts. The rash is mildly pruritic and scaly. It is present on his cheek, back and neck, but does not extend to his face, legs, hands or feet.

1. Based on the history and physical examination, your diagnosis is:
   A. Nummular eczema
   B. Syphilis
   C. Pityriasis rosea
   D. Tinea versicolor
   E. Psoriasis

2. The most important test to perform on this patient is:
   A. Skin culture
   B. KOH preparation
   C. Serum RPR
   D. Skin biopsy
   E. None of the above

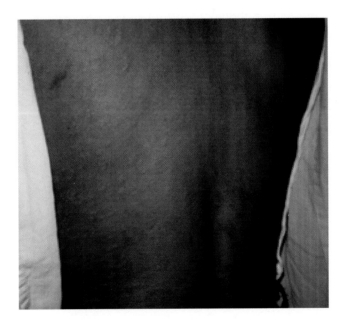

DISCUSSION

ANSWERS:
1. C. Pityriasis rosea
2. C. Serum RPR

1. The rash is that of pityriasis rosa, a papulosquamous eruption that often begins with a "herald patch" and then evolves into a series of silvery, ovoid-shaped plaques that appear in horizontal planes on the trunk, back and neck. This accounts for the so-called "Christmas tree" pattern of distribution. Secondary syphilis may have an identical appearance, but it is far less common in adolescents. Other rashes to considered in the differential diagnosis include drug reactions, Mucha-Habermann disease, seborrheic dermatitis, nummular eczema, and guttate psoriasis.

   The "herald patch" occurs in 80% of children and may be mistaken for a lesion of tinea corporis or a patch of nummular eczema. These lesions have their own characteristic morphology, rather than being papulosquamous, and are much fewer in number. Tinea versicolor is characterized by flat areas of hypo- and hyperpigmentation.

2. The most important test to be performed is an RPR, as secondary syphilis can mimic pityriasis rosa. In this patient who is sexually active, it is important to rule out syphilis, even when the rash is entirely consistent with pityriasis rosa. KOH serves to identify *Pityrosporum obiculare*, the cause of tinea versicolor. Skin culture may be useful for lesions that do not have a completely characteristic morphology but are suspected to be infectious in origin. Although useful for difficult to diagnose chronic disorders, rarely is skin biopsy indicated for an acute dermatitis.

Further Discussion

The etiology of pityriasis rosa remains unknown; thus, the treatment is symptomatic. Antihistamines will help with the pruritus, as will topical emollients. Many patients of their own initiative engage in frequent washing when a rash appears. With pityriasis rosa, drying of the skin will cause more pruritus. Mild soaps and infrequent bathing are suggested.

CASE 115

An 11-year-old girl complains of abdominal pain for 4 days, fever, nonbilious vomiting, and nonbloody, watery stools. For the past 2 days, she has refused to take anything by mouth. She has no medical problems and has never been hospitalized. Her temperature is 39°C, and she is tachycardic to 140/min. Her physical examination is notable for diffuse tenderness in the lower abdomen without rebound. You order intravenous fluids, laboratory studies, and X-rays.

1. The most likely diagnosis is:
    A. Bacterial gastroenteritis
    B. Midgut volvulus
    C. Acute appendicitis
    D. Intra-abdominal abscess
    E. Meckel's diverticulum

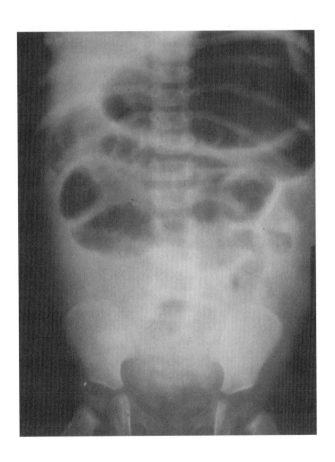

DISCUSSION

ANSWER:

1. **D. Intra-abdominal abscess**

1. This girl has an appendiceal (intra-abdominal) abscess, rather than acute appendicitis, based on the duration of her history, the examination of her abdomen, and her X-rays. One needs to be wary about the diagnosis of bacterial enteritis in this patient with 4 days of abdominal pain and high fever but no bloody stools, who in addition has a fecalith. A midgut volvulus occurs less often than appendicitis at this age and would not be associated with a fecalith. Although an inflamed Meckel's diverticulum can mimic appendicitis, it is also much less common.

Further Discussion

Appendicitis represents the most common surgical emergency in children. The highest incidence occurs between the ages of 10 and 19 years. Children also have the highest perforation rate. The process begins with obstruction of the appendiceal lumen by fecal material or inflamed lymphoid tissue. The patient experiences vague epigastric pain, resulting from referred impulses along the nerves in the T 10 and T 11 dermatomes. Lymphatic obstruction and venous congestion of the appendix follow, resulting in ischemia. Pain then localizes in the right lower quadrant due to peritoneal inflammation. Eventually, arterial blood flow is compromised and perforation occurs, producing the signs of diffuse peritonitis. Transient improvement may be noted at the time of rupture. If a perforation is contained locally, the patient may not manifest the usual findings of a ruptured appendix.

Appendicitis can mimic many intra-abdominal processes. Additionally, some patients may begin with gastroenteritis and develop appendicitis subsequently, after having been correctly diagnosed with a nonsurgical process at the first visit. There is virtually no symptom which rules out the diagnosis. The majority of patients have abdominal pain that is followed by anorexia and vomiting. Five to 10% have diarrhea. Most series of laparotomies for possible appendicitis include 10 to 30% of cases with a normal appendix.

Findings on the plain radiograph are usually non-specific, but may be abnormal in approximately 35% of patients. Early on, in the presence of anorexia and vomiting, the abdomen will be airless. Occasionally, lumbar scoliosis is seen due to spasm of the overlying rectus abdominal muscles in the presence of peritoneal inflammation. In 20-30% of patients, a fecalith may be seen in the right lower quadrant. This is due to inspissated, calcified feces in the appendix. With perforation and abscess formation, there may be absence of air in the right lower quadrant or organized "step ladder" loops of bowel consistent with a mechanical small bowel obstruction. Free air is a late sign of perforation. Since the majority of patients in whom the diagnosis is made at laparotomy have non specific radiographic findings, the history and physical examination are the most important components of the evaluation.

In this patient, a fecalith is seen in the right lower quadrant. Additionally, she has a paucity of air in the right lower quadrant with dilated proximal loops and little distal air, suggestive of a partial small bowel obstruction. On the decubitus view (see figure on next page), air fluid levels are readily noted, a finding that is also consistent with ileus.

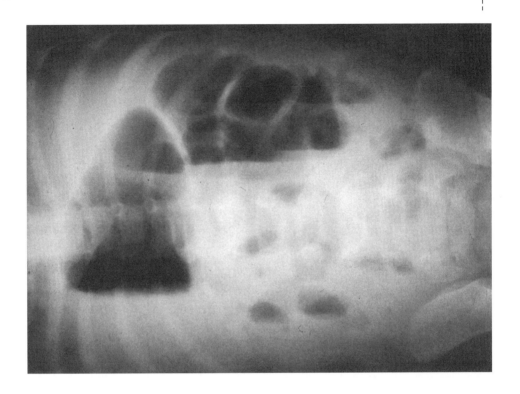

An 18-month-old is brought to the emergency department with a blistering rash in the diaper area. The mother reports that she just noticed it today, and that the child has been otherwise well. The child's past medical history is negative except for 3 or 4 ear infections. His vital signs are: P 120/min, R 28/min, BP 105/55 mm Hg, and T 38.0°C. He has fluid behind both tympanic membranes and mild rhinorrhea. The remainder of the examination is normal except as shown.

1. Your provisional diagnosis is:
    A. Child abuse
    B. Staphylococcal scalded skin syndrome
    C. Chemical dermatitis
    D. Bullous impetigo
    E. Bullous pemphigus

2. Based on your impression you would:
    A. Culture the nares
    B. Do a Gram stain
    C. Measure skin pH
    D. Do a skin biopsy
    E. File an abuse report

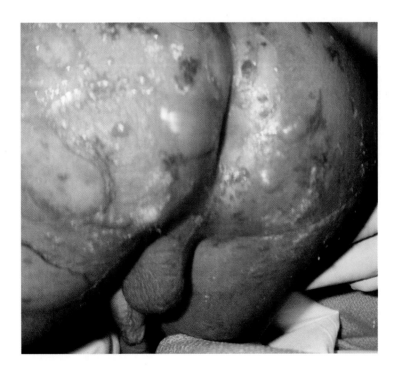

DISCUSSION

ANSWERS:
1. A. Child abuse
2. E. File an abuse report

1. Skin loss and blistering over this amount of the body surface area is most likely the result of thermal injury; given the history, or lack thereof, and the distribution of involvement, child abuse is the correct answer. Staphylococcal scalded skin syndrome (SSSS) is a toxin-mediated disorder in which there is cleavage of the skin at the epidermal level. This is never just confined to one area of the body. It is characterized by diffuse erythema followed by peeling that can be produced by minor trauma, such as rubbing (Nikolsky Sign). The staphylococci may be in the nose or elsewhere in the body. Chemical burns of the buttocks may occur if the parent has inappropriately used an acidic or alkaline product on the skin. In such cases, the history is usually evident. Bullous impetigo can cause a blistering rash, but never over such a widespread area nor to this depth; the onset is usually gradual with spread occurring over several days to a week. Bullous pemphigoid is a rare, chronic bullous disease.

2. To further evaluate your clinical suspicions, you should file a report of suspected abuse. As mentioned above, culture of the nares may yield staphylococci in patients with scalded skin syndrome. If a chemical cause is suspected, measuring the pH of the skin is appropriate and rinsing until the pH is normal is the best initial treatment. With impetigo, a Gram stain and culture of a lesion would be diagnostic. A skin biopsy is useful for the diagnosis of bullous pemphigus.

Further Discussion

Immersion burns are a common form of child abuse. When parents have unrealistic expectations about the ability of their child to learn toilet training, they may become convinced that the child is having "accidents" as an act of defiance. In part to clean the child and in part to punish, they may submerge the buttocks in hot water producing first and second degree burns. In many residential locations, hot water heaters can produce water at 140° F. Even brief exposure to water at that temperature will produce thermal injury.

The red hue noted in some localized areas of this child's burn was caused when the mother applied tomato paste to the burn area with the thought that this was appropriate first aid.

A 4-month-old boy is brought to the emergency department by his mother who states that he has been increasingly irritable over the past 24 hours. This morning he vomited a couple of times and since then she has offered him Pedialyte®, which he has taken slowly. There is no history of fever, upper respiratory tract symptoms, diarrhea, or rash. His last bowel movement was 2 days ago, which is a normal pattern for him. He was born after a 31-week gestation at a birth weight of 1800 grams and had an uncomplicated 2-week hospitalization for feeding and growing. On physical examination, he is afebrile with stable vital signs. He is remarkably irritable, and he has a distended abdomen. It is impossible to assess pain to palpation or bowel sounds because of his crying. You proceed with screening laboratory tests and an abdominal film.

1. Your diagnosis is:
    A. Meckel's diverticulum
    B. Pyloric stenosis
    C. Duodenal atresia
    D. Inguinal hernia
    E. Gastroenteritis

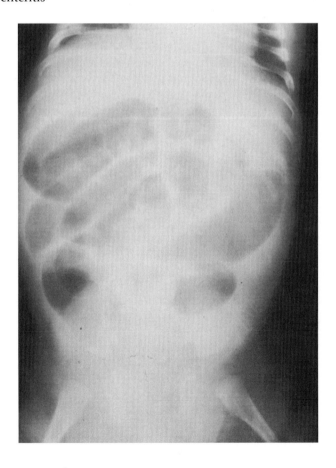

DISCUSSION

ANSWER:

1. D. Inguinal hernia

1. This child has an incarcerated inguinal hernia, causing a mechanical obstruction, as seen on his X-ray which shows distended loops of bowel with little distal air and some accentuation of the soft tissues in the left inguinal region. Although air may be seen sometimes in the hernia sac, this was not the case here. Duodenal atresia usually manifests in the first 2 days of life and causes a high obstruction that produces a "double bubble" sign. Pyloric stenosis affects infants between 3 and 8 weeks of age. Radiographically, one may see a distended stomach and a relatively gasless abdomen but not a picture consistent with a small bowel obstruction. Meckel's diverticulum generally presents with painless rectal bleeding, most often at 2 years of age, and it may also cause a syndrome similar to appendicitis. Although gastroenteritis is common, one must be wary of making this diagnosis in a child with vomiting who has no fever or diarrhea. In this instance, the physician correctly pursued a mechanical etiology for the vomiting and obtained an X-ray, which is not compatible with an infectious etiology for the vomiting.

Further Discussion

Incarcerated inguinal hernias are the most common cause of bowel obstruction in the first year of life. The true incidence of inguinal hernias is unknown, but they are estimated to occur at a rate of 10-20/1000 live births. Inguinal hernias are found more commonly in boys, usually on the right side; 60% of incarcerated hernias occur in the first year of life.

Inguinal hernias are most often diagnosed by the parent or caretaker after a bulge is noted in the child's groin. Most patients are otherwise asymptomatic, unless incarceration occurs. Irritability, abdominal distension and occasionally vomiting are seen with incarcerated hernias. The diagnosis of a hernia is difficult, if a bulge is not present during the physical examination. Maneuvers to increase intra-abdominal pressure, such as restraining the infant's legs and arms while lying on the examination table, may cause the hernia sac to fill. The physician should also look for thickening of the cord by placing the index finger over the area of the cord at the pubic space. While gently rubbing back and forth, the walls of the sac rub against each other, producing the "silk sign," the sensation of two pieces of silk rubbing together. Transillumination is of limited value.

In patients with incarcerated inguinal hernias, the abdominal radiograph most often reveals evidence of small bowel obstruction. Air may or may not be seen in the hernia sac. One may also see prominence of the inguinal soft tissue fold on the affected side.

Children presenting with reducible inguinal hernias may be referred for outpatient surgical repair. Reduction should be attempted in children presenting with incarcerated hernias as long as there is no evidence of gangrenous bowel. With patience, and sometimes with sedation, 80% of these are reducible. Following reduction, the hernia is electively repaired once swelling of the tissues has resolved, greatly reducing the complication rate.

A 12-year-old complains of a rash around one of his eyes. He states that it is intensely pruritic. He has had a mild upper respiratory infection for several days, but no fever. His history is unremarkable except for "itchy" skin and occasional rashes since infancy.

1. Your diagnosis is
    A. Herpes zoster
    B. Periorificial dermatitis
    C. Bullous impetigo
    D. Eczema herpeticum
    E. Atopic dermatitis

2. You prescribe:
    A. Acyclovir
    B. Cephalexin
    C. Mupirocin
    D. Tetracycline
    E. Hydrocortisone

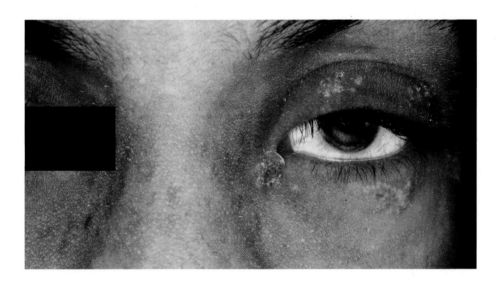

DISCUSSION

ANSWERS:
1. D. Eczema herpeticum
2. A. Acyclovir

1. The diagnosis is eczema herpeticum, as one sees vesicles superimposed on a background of eczematous skin. Most likely, the virus spread from an asymptomatic gingivostomatitis. This eruption could be easily confused with zoster, which is unilateral and often occurs along the ophthalmic branch of the trigeminal nerve. However, the lesions are localized rather than dermatomal and, with zoster, the adjacent skin would be normal rather than eczematous. Periorificial dermatitis usually occurs around both eyes and the mouth; the lesions are scaly, but neither eczematous nor vesicular. In bullous impetigo, the vesicles generally vary considerably in size and appear purulent. Finally, atopic dermatitis is characterized by lichenification and eczematous changes in the skin, but not by vesicles, unless superinfected.

2. Acyclovir is effective against Herpes simplex virus. Either oral cephalexin or topical mupirocin represent reasonable choices for bullous impetigo. Tetracycline is recommended for periorificial dermatitis, and hydrocortisone for atopic dermatitis.

Further Discussion

Vesicular lesions around the eye raise the specter of herpetic keratitis. In this patient, one would want to perform fluorescein staining of the cornea, looking for a dendritic ulcer. Topical antiviral therapy and care by an ophthalmologist are recommended for herpetic keratitis, but prophylactic therapy is not routinely prescribed when lesions occur near the eye.

A 3-year-old arrives via an ambulance, immobilized on a posterior spine board. He was riding in a car involved in a motor vehicle collision, while traveling at an estimated speed of 50 mph. His mother, the driver, is badly injured. Although restrained in a car seat, the seat itself was not belted in place. The child was found in the front seat, in the car seat, crying furiously. On physical examination, his vital signs are within normal limits. He has a contusion on the center of his forehead. He appears to be moving all of his extremities symmetrically. His initial lateral cervical radiograph appears below.

1. You diagnose a:
   A. Hangman's fracture
   B. Jefferson fracture
   C. Burst fracture
   D. Dens fracture
   E. Tear drop fracture

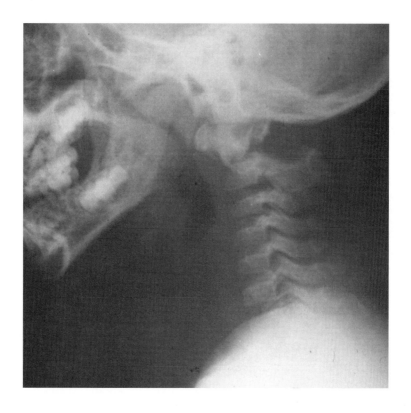

DISCUSSION

ANSWER:

1. **D. Dens fracture**

1. This lateral view demonstrates a fracture at the base of the dens with anterior dislocation. A Hangman's fracture is characterized by bilateral fractures of C2 pedicles and dislocation of C2 on C3. The postulated mechanism is hyperextension as the rope becomes taught, followed by flexion. In a Jefferson fracture, the atlas bursts, and one sees symmetrical bilateral displacement of its articular masses over the edge of the axis. Both wedge and burst fractures affect the vertebral bodies. The wedge fracture is caused by mechanical compression of the involved vertebra during forceful flexion. Although there is no fracture line, the vertebra exhibits a loss of stature. By way of contrast, a burst fracture is characterized by a vertical fracture line and the vertebral body is comminuted.

Further Discussion

In children, there is a synchondrosis at the base of the dens that disappears between the ages of 5 and 7 years. Do not mistake this for a fracture when viewing lateral cervical spine films. Fractures of the dens result from flexion injuries and are typically associated with anterior displacement. When viewing the lateral film, in the normal situation, the dens tilts posteriorly. When a fracture occurs, there is anterior tilting of the dens, which may be the only evidence that a fracture occurs on the plain film. In this child, the anterior displacement is very clearly seen. The predental space, that space between the dens and the anterior arch of C1, remains normal. The transverse and alar ligaments responsible for holding the dens within the ring if C1 remain intact, and thus these two elements have moved together. Nondisplaced fractures through the base of the dens may go undetected unless a CT scan is obtained or subsequent films at a later date reveal bony resorption.

A 9-year-old, previously healthy boy complains of a rash for 2 days, One week after returning from summer camp, he developed of a headache and was noted to have a low grade fever. On the next day, a rash began as shown. On examination, he has a temperature of 38.5°C, a pulse of 120/min, respirations of 22/min, and a blood pressure of 105/75 mm Hg. He does not have photophobia, conjunctivitis, or nuchal rigidity.

1. Your treatment for this infection is:
   A. Erythromycin
   B. Acetaminophen
   C. Ceftriaxone
   D. Tetracycline
   E. Penicillin

2. A likely abnormality is:
   A. Na 128 mEq/L
   B. HCO_3 12 mEq/L
   C. Platelets 850,000/mm^3
   D. BUN 65 mg/dl
   E. Hct 18%

3. Laboratory confirmation of your diagnosis might be provided by:
   A. RPR
   B. Viral cultures
   C. Complement fixation titers
   D. Blood culture
   E. Cerebrospinal fluid culture

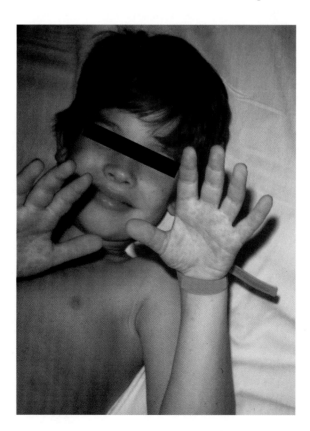

DISCUSSION

ANSWERS:
1. D. Tetracycline
2. A. Na 128 mEq/L
3. C. Complement fixation titers

1. This boy has Rocky Mountain spotted fever (RMSF). The antibiotics of choice are tetracycline and chloramphenicol. Tetracycline is relatively contraindicated in children less than 8 years of age, due to the possibility that it may stain the dentition. Another infection that causes a rash on the palms and soles is syphilis, but the age of the patient and the epidemiology make this condition highly unlikely. Syphilis is treated with benzathine penicillin. If one suspected meningococcemia, ceftriaxone would be an excellent choice. The eruption of meningococcemia is often petechial from the outset, does not particularly involve the palms and soles, and generally would cause the patient to be at least somewhat ill appearing. Erythromycin is the drug of choice for mycoplasmal disease and acetaminophen would suffice for a viral infection, such as Coxsackie hand-foot-mouth disease.

2. Hyponatremia and thrombocytopenia, as opposed to thrombocytosis, may occur with RMSF. This child appears relatively well, but severely ill patients with RMSF, or meningococcemia, may develop acidosis and anemia, on the basis of disseminated intravascular coagulation. Marked elevation of the BUN characterizes hemolytic uremic syndrome.

3. The most accurate test to diagnosis RMSF is a specific serological assay, such as complement fixation or microimmunofluorescence. Cross reacting antibodies to *Proteus*, the Weil Felix test, are neither sensitive nor specific and have fallen out of favor. If meningococcemia were suspected, cultures of the blood and cerebrospinal fluid would be indicated. The RPR tests for syphilis.

Further Discussion

RMSF is caused by *Rickettsia rickettsii* and transmitted by dog and wood ticks. The incubation period is 2-10 days, which fits with the appearance of the first symptoms approximately one week after returning from summer camp. Fever and headache herald the onset of RMSF, followed by a maculopapular rash, which usually begins on the wrists and ankle and spreads quickly to the palms and soles. After 1-3 days, the rash becomes petechial. Many patients with RMSF respond to oral antibiotic therapy as outpatients, when the diagnosis is made early the course before the onset of coagulopathy.

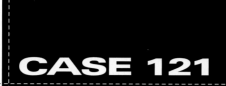

A father brings his son to the emergency department after he noticed "blood in his eye."

1. The most common therapy for this lesion is:
   A. Eye shield
   B. Topical anesthetics
   C. Eye patch
   D. Topical antimicrobials
   E. None of the above

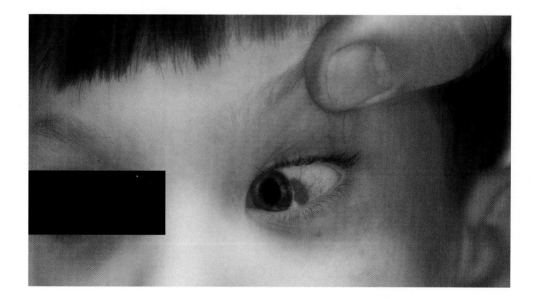

DISCUSSION

ANSWER:

1. **E. None of the above**

1. This patient has a sharply demarcated red area on his bulbar conjunctiva most consistent with a subconjunctival hemorrhage. None of the therapies should be recommended since the hemorrhage will resolve over the next 2-3 weeks. An eye shield should be used for any child who has evidence of ruptured globe, which should be suspected after trauma leading to a 360° subconjunctival hemorrhage around the cornea. Topical anesthetics have a short duration of action and are only used in the emergency setting to allow a more complete examination of the patient. Eye patches provide some relief for a child with a corneal abrasion, but not for subconjunctival hemorrhage. Topical antibiotics are used to treat bacterial infections, which would appear as more diffuse conjunctival injection with a purulent exudate.

Further Discussion

Subconjunctival hemorrhage can be seen after increased intrathoracic pressure due to trauma, or associated with blood dyscrasias, hypertension, or infection. Probably the most common precipitant is increased orbital venous pressure due to coughing (e.g., pertussis) or vomiting. The small red areas around this patient's orbit might be periorbital petechiae, another common finding after severe coughing or vomiting.

A 12-week-old infant is brought to the emergency department by his mother because he has not been moving his legs for the past 2 days. The mother gives no history of trauma or fever. He was born at term; pregnancy and delivery were uncomplicated. His mother thinks that his face looks puffy. On physical examination he appears thin and has mild peri-orbital edema and hepatosplenomegaly. Although you cannot appreciate any obvious swelling or focal tenderness, he cries when his legs are moved.

1. After reviewing the radiographs you decide to do the following:
    A. Call the child abuse team
    B. Order a calcium and phosphorus
    C. Obtain a blood culture
    D. Draw an RPR titer
    E. Send a hemoglobin electrophoresis

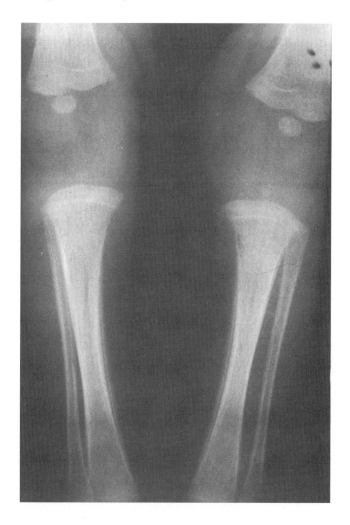

DISCUSSION

ANSWER:

1. **D. Draw an RPR titer**

1. This infant has the typical bony lesions and periosteal elevation seen with syphilis, which is diagnosed by an elevated RPR titer. If you saw periosteal reaction and callous formation secondary to multiple fractures of different ages, filing a report of child abuse would be appropriate. However, in this example, the reaction is too diffuse and there is evidence of bony destruction. Calcium and phosphorus levels are abnormal in rickets; typical findings on X-ray include osteopenia and ragged, concave epiphyses. Oxacillin is often chosen to treat osteomyelitis, caused most often by *Staphylococcus aureus*. Radiographic changes of osteomyelitis are not seen until 10-14 days into the disease and appear as lytic lesions and/or a periosteal reaction, generally at a single focus. Patients with sickle cell disease, diagnosed definitively with hemoglobin electrophoresis, may have also have lytic lesions and/or periosteal new bone formation due to old infarcts. This child is too young to have bony changes from sickle cell anemia, as he would have predominantly fetal hemoglobin in his circulation.

Further Discussion

The majority of patients with congenital syphilis develop symptoms within the first 3 months of life, and over two-thirds of these infants have osteochondritis and/or periostitis. Multiple, symmetrical bony changes are seen in areas of rapid growth on the radiographs. Bones of the lower extremities are most commonly involved, particularly the tibia, but the upper extremity may be affected frequently as well. Disease is often localized to the metaphysis and seen as broad areas of radiolucency or focal destructive lesions. Diaphyseal involvement manifests as periosteal elevation due to new bone formation.

This patient presented with pseudoparalysis of Parrot due to epiphysitis resulting in pain with movement of the joints of the lower extremities. Interestingly, the swelling that his mother noted was due to nephrotic syndrome, a manifestation of congenital syphilis. In this child's X-rays, periosteal elevation is seen throughout. In the radiograph of the upper extremity (see figure below), the diaphysis has a mottled appearance and there is radiolucency of the distal humerus and extensive periosteal new bone formation. In the lower extremities, there is bilateral periosteal elevation. Also note the growth arrest lines in all of the long bones. These radiographic findings are diagnostic of syphilis.

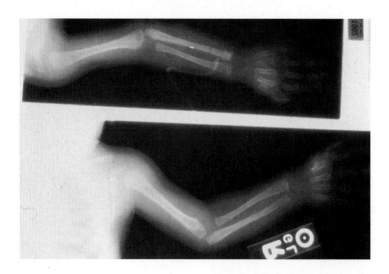

A 4-year-old boy is brought to the emergency department by his parents. They state that he was well until 3-4 days ago when he developed some sores on his chest that they thought were insect bites. The lesions have spread and scabbed. Now the child has developed a rash and fever. The parents have noted peeling skin around his mouth and nose. When they touch his skin, it rubs off in sheets.

1. Based on these findings, you would diagnose:
    A. Toxic shock syndrome
    B. Stevens-Johnson syndrome
    C. Staphylococcal scalded skin syndrome
    D. Scarlet fever
    E. Kawasaki disease

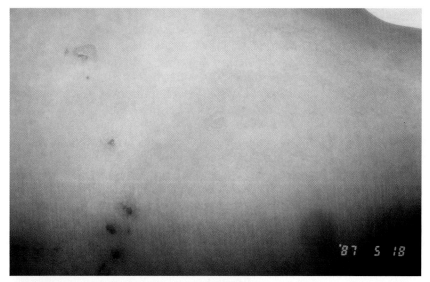

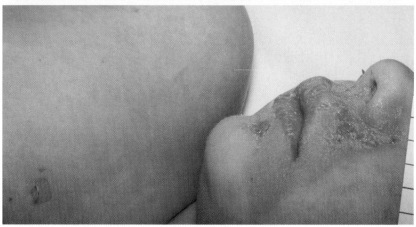

DISCUSSION

ANSWER:

1. C. Staphylococcal scalded skin syndrome

1. The findings are typical for staphylococcal scalded skin syndrome (SSSS). Although it can cause large areas of denuded skin and excess fluid loss leading to mild dehydration, SSSS is not associated with the systemic circulatory failure noted in toxic shock syndrome. Stevens-Johnson syndrome (SJS) is marked by mucous membrane involvement as a dominant feature. SJS is usually triggered by a drug exposure or by a herpes virus or other infection. The eruption may be maculopapular or vesicular-bullous. Scarlet fever, caused by *Streptococcus pyogenes*, is characterized by a sandpapery rash, accentuated in the antecubital folds (Pastia's lines). Desquamation occurs as a late finding, but affected patients do not have a positive Nikolsky's sign. Kawasaki disease is similar to SSSS and scarlet fever in that it is a toxin-mediated condition. In addition to a rash, one observes persistent fever, conjunctivitis, mucositis, and cervical lymphadenopathy.

Further Discussion

Staphylococcal scalded skin syndrome results from either a staphylococcal infection or benign carriage of the organism. Staphylococci are usually not recovered from the blood or from an aspirate of an intact bullous lesion. With careful culturing, the organism may be found in the nares or at the base of the scabbed lesions. Bacteria have also been isolated from the eyes, rectum, throat and vagina in some cases. The first clinical signs are fever, malaise and irritability. There is diffuse erythema or a sunburn appearance of the skin. The skin is very tender to palpation, and sheets of skin may peel with gentle traction (Nikolsky's sign). The patient may develop vesicles, pustules or bullae. Frequently there is a purulent drainage from the eyes but no true conjunctivitis. The mucous membranes are not involved in SSSS, as in SJS. Management of children with SSSS includes admission to the hospital and administration of an anti-staphylococcal antibiotic intravenously. The use of steroids is discouraged. The physician must pay close attention to fluid and electrolyte balance, particularly in the young child where there is an increased surface area-to-weight ratio. Secondary infections may develop.

This 5-year-old girl is brought to the emergency department with a 3-week history of "allergic" eyes and a 1 week history of weight gain and malaise. Her vital signs are normal. Positive findings on examination are seen in the photographs

1. Which of the following tests is most likely to appropriately narrow the differential diagnosis?
   A. Bilirubin, ALT, and AST
   B. Urine dipstick
   C. Total protein and albumin
   D. Electrolytes, BUN, creatinine
   E. Chest X-ray

2. After the laboratory studies return, the vital signs are unchanged, but the child is very uncomfortable due to the edema. Initial management might begin with:
   A. Normal saline, 20 cc/kg, IV
   B. Oral fluids at twice maintenance
   C. A trial of diuretics
   D. Intravenous antibiotics
   E. Cyclophosphamide

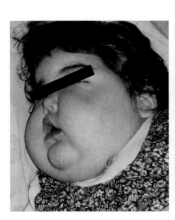
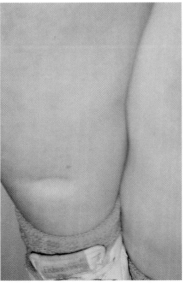
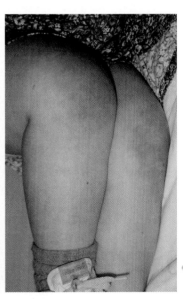

DISCUSSION

ANSWERS:
1. **B. Urine dipstick**
2. **C. A trial of diuretics**

1. The photographs show a child with generalized edema, most pronounced either in areas that are very distensible, such as her eyes and face, or dependent regions, like her legs. Life-threatening causes of generalized edema need to be rapidly confirmed or excluded. Generalized edema is usually caused by cardiac, renal, hepatic, or allergic disease. Congestive heart failure or pericardial disease that is severe enough to cause generalized edema in a child should lead to tachycardia, tachypnea, and an S3 gallop. An allergic reaction usually causes localized edema, often with urticaria. Hepatic failure can cause generalized edema, but is more likely to present as jaundice in a child. Renal disease, with proteinuria and hypoalbuminemia, is the most common etiology for generalized edema in childhood. The quickest way to narrow the diagnostic possibilities would be a urine dipstick to evaluate for proteinuria, a 60-second test, which suggests nephrotic syndrome, when positive. Hematuria on the dipstick would be less common and point to glomerulonephritis. Decreased serum total protein and albumin, in association with proteinuria, would confirm the diagnosis of nephrotic syndrome, but, in isolation, are not specific. Electrolytes, BUN and creatinine need to be checked, but could be abnormal in renal, cardiac, or hepatic disease. A chest X-ray would be helpful if you strongly suspected congestive heart failure, and might also show a pleural effusion associated with nephrotic syndrome. In the absence of jaundice or a history of hepatic disease, liver function tests are unlikely to be useful.

2. Although patients with nephrotic syndrome are edematous, they are not usually intravascularly fluid overloaded, and may even be hypovolemic or even in shock. However with normal vital signs this patient does not appear to be in shock and should not receive 20 cc/kg of intravenous normal saline. If she appeared more mildly dehydrated, oral fluids could be tried. Since she is well hydrated but very uncomfortable, a trial of diuretics would be an excellent choice for initial management. Antibiotics should be withheld unless the patient had signs of infection. Immunosuppressants, such as cyclophosphamide, are not the initial therapeutic agents in nephrotic syndrome.

Further Discussion

Nephrotic syndrome is a relatively common occurrence in children between 1 and 4 years of age. The vast majority are classified as "nil change" nephrosis, meaning that the histology of the kidneys is relatively normal. The likelihood of "nil change" is sufficiently high at that age that generally treatment is instituted without performing a biopsy. The initial therapy consists primarily of corticosteroids. Patients with refractory disease may require treatment with more potent immunosuppressive agents, such as cyclophosphamide, and biopsy. Children with nephrosis may develop complications necessitating emergency intervention. Despite the total body fluid overload, intravascular depletion may occur. Other complications include thromboses and primary bacterial peritonitis.

A 2-year-old child has had high fever and cough for 2 days. Upon arrival to the emergency department, she is cyanotic and aerating her lungs poorly. You intubate her trachea without difficulty and administer 100% oxygen, leading to a saturation of 95%. As the technologist enters the room pushing a portable X-ray machine, the saturation monitor alarms and the child again appears blue. Her pulse is 180/min and her blood pressure is 50 mm Hg by palpation. Her breath sounds are equal.

1. As a next step you would:
   A. Give a saline bolus over 20 minutes
   B. Needle both hemithoraces
   C. Begin a dopamine infusion
   D. Replace the endotracheal tube
   E. Perform pericardiocentesis

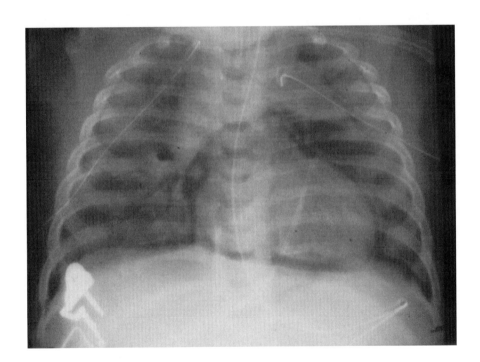

DISCUSSION

ANSWERS:

1. **E. Perform pericardiocentesis**

1. This is an example of a pneumopericardium, which is under tension based on the clinical deterioration and the vital signs, and must be evacuated by pericardiocentesis. Volume infusion provides temporary relief from hypotension in some cases of tamponade, but it would be poor practice to rely on fluid administration alone for 20 minutes in this case. Other potential causes for clinical deterioration include an endotracheal tube that has become either blocked or displaced, a tension pneumothorax, and septic shock. Although it is appropriate in some instances to blindly "needle" both hemithoraces, this X-ray excludes a pneumothorax. Given that the breath sounds are equal bilaterally and the endotracheal tube appears to be properly positioned radiographically, re-intubating the child in not necessary and might prove disastrous. Septic shock with a bacterial pneumonia could well cause hypotension in this patient, but would be unlikely to produce a sudden, life-threatening change in her condition. Both volume infusion and dopamine are appropriate therapies in septic shock.

Further Discussion

With pneumopericardium, a continuous radiolucent border surrounds the heart, including the lower margin just above the diaphragm. If a fine white line is visualized, representing the pericardium as it is separated away from the heart by air, then the diagnosis is cinched. Air is not seen lateral to the great vessels, a finding that distinguishes pneumopericardium from pneumomediastinum. Barotrauma to an injured lung is the most common cause of pneumopericardium.

The hypotension in this patient is due to impingement on cardiac filling. Therapy is aimed at overcoming the impediment to cardiac filling with volume infusion and evacuation of the air in the pericardial space. Clinically, it may be difficult to differentiate pneumothorax, pneumomediastinum or pneumopericardium. A pneumothorax would be a more common cause of deterioration in an intubated patient on positive pressure ventilation, and an absence of or decreased breath sounds on the involved side is a common physical finding. Pneumomediastinum infrequently creates significant tension and cardiovascular compromise, as the air can decompress into the extra-thoracic soft tissues.

A 14-year-old boy sustained a laceration over his lower extremity while trying to scale a metal fence approximately 5 hours ago.

1. Closure of this wound will be facilitated by:
    A. Debridement to create an ellipse
    B. Application of tissue adhesive
    C. Placement of a skin graft
    D. Use of half-buried mattress sutures
    E. Extensive undermining of the wound

2. Despite an excellent repair using chromic sutures in the subcutaneous tissues, this wound may undergo a dehiscence because:
    A. The boy waited too long before seeking treatment
    B. Synthetic sutures should have been used, not chromic
    C. Metal is more likely than wood to cause an infection
    D. After the age of 6 years, tissues heal less readily
    E. The wound is adjacent to a joint

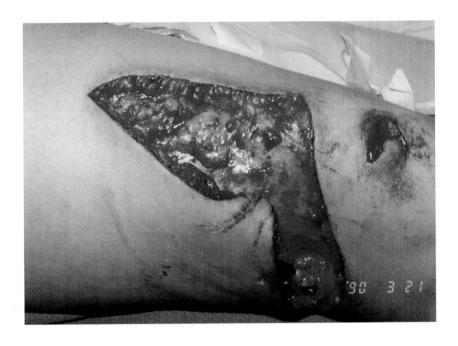

DISCUSSION

ANSWERS:

1. **D. Use of half-buried mattress sutures**
2. **E. The wound is adjacent to a joint**

1. This wound has a triangular flap. While the broad, proximal base of the flap favors a successful repair, one still wants to maximize circulation to the tip. Placement of one or more half-buried mattress sutures helps to accomplish this goal. Both extensive debridement and grafting are completely unnecessary. Primary repair is preferable to debridement and more likely to produce an acceptable cosmetic result in this situation. Although it may appear to the inexperienced observer that tissue has been avulsed, this is not the case. Rather, the flap has retracted, as expected; it can be advanced by placement of subcuticular sutures. Extensive undermining is not needed and will only further compromise the blood supply. The wound is too large to allow for a tissue adhesive.

2. Location on the extensor surface adjacent to the knee predisposes this laceration to dehiscence. Generally, extremity wounds heal well if repaired in the first 8-12 hours, so the boy did not wait too long. Neither synthetic nor chromic sutures predispose a wound to dehiscence. While the circulation is compromised in old age, this is not an issue in a 14-year-old boy. Organic material, such as wood (as opposed to metal), may lead to retained foreign bodies and infection.

Further Discussion

This is a challenging laceration, given the location and the mild delay in seeking treatment. To begin, it should be copiously irrigated. Conservative debridement of devitalized tissue would be appropriate. After a meticulous layered closure, I would immobilize the extremity with a posterior splint and recommend elevation for 48 hours.

A 10-year-old male is brought to the emergency department with a painful finger for the last 3 days. He is afebrile.

1. Definitive therapy for this lesion is:
   A. Oral antistaphylococcal antibiotics
   B. Topical antibiotics
   C. Incision between eponychium and nail bed.
   D. Finger pad incision with wick placement
   E. Warm soaks

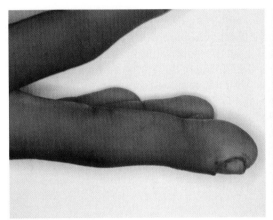
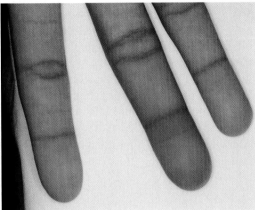

DISCUSSION

ANSWER:

1. D. Incision between eponychium and nail bed

1. The eponychium is elevated and pale due to a collection of pus between it and the nail root. The nails are very short, suggesting that the child bites his nails. Although this infection is likely to caused by *Staphylococcus aureus* or *Streptococcus pyogenes*, systemic antibiotics will not treat it once a collection of pus has formed. If the area were not fluctuant, warm soaks might help localize the infection and then allow definitive therapy. Topical antibiotics are adequate for impetigo, but not a pus collection. This abscess, a paronychia, will require an incision between the eponychium and the nail bed to drain the pus. An incision of the finger pad would be therapeutic for a felon, an abscess of the pulp space on the ventral aspect of the distal phalanx. In a felon, the pulp of the finger is very red, swollen and extremely tender. The eponychium should be normal.

Further Discussion

After anesthetizing the finger with a digital nerve block and prepping the tip, sweep a #11 blade through the space between the nail bed and the eponychium, keeping the blade parallel to the nail plate. A small wick can be placed under the eponychium to promote drainage for the first 24 to 48 hours. When the drain is removed at 24 to 48 hours, the patient is instructed to soak the finger in warm water 3 times a day to keep the wound open and draining. If the pus collection has extended under the nail, a portion of the nail may need to be removed. In cases with a surrounding area of cellulitis or lymphangitic streaking, systemic antibiotics may hasten the resolution.

A 12-month-old boy is brought for evaluation of a swollen eye. His mother states that she noticed it last evening and today it seems worse. She gave him acetaminophen last night for a fever. There has been no drainage from the eye, but he has had an upper respiratory tract infection over the past week or two. He is otherwise healthy and has received his immunizations. Currently, he has a temperature of 40°C and appears nontoxic.

1. The most likely cause of this child's eye swelling is:
   A. Sinusitis
   B. Unrecognized trauma
   C. Preseptal cellulitis
   D. Bacterial conjunctivitis
   E. Orbital cellulitis

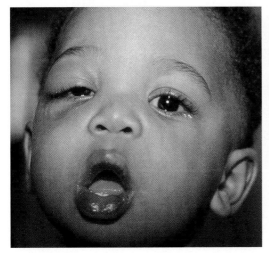
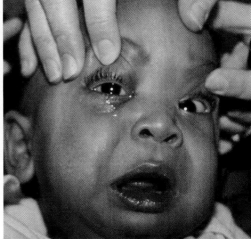

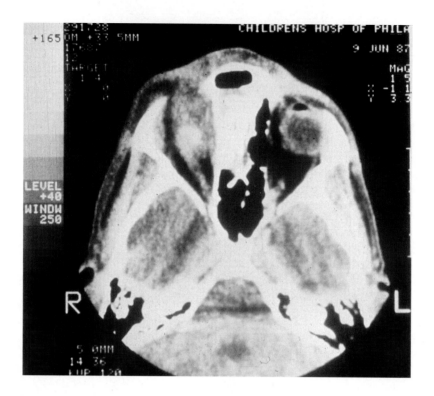

DISCUSSION

ANSWER:

1. E. Orbital cellulitis

1. This child has orbital cellulitis, an infection of the space behind the orbital septum, which is bounded by the ethmoid, maxillary and frontal sinuses. In the first picture, swelling surrounding the right eye is noted with a small amount of erythema. In the second picture, note limitation of abduction of the right eye. The orbital CAT scan reveals edema and abscess formation in the ocular muscles along with mild proptosis of the right eye.

Further Discussion

Clinically, it can be difficult to distinguish orbital from preseptal cellulitis, which is an infection of the space anterior to the orbital septum. Preseptal involvement is more common in young children and often results from bacteremia or microtrauma with secondary infection. Both orbital and preseptal cellulitis cause swelling around the eye and fever. In preseptal cellulitis, the typical characteristics of cellulitis are present including erythema, induration, swelling, warmth, and tenderness to palpation. Conjunctival involvement is rare, ocular mobility and vision are normal, and there is no proptosis. Orbital cellulitis results from direct extension of a sinus infection from the sinus to the orbit, most commonly through the lamina papyracea. Limited external ocular movements are often seen in these patients due to edema of the eye muscles and/or abscess formation. Proptosis may be appreciated on physical examination and vision may impaired. Chemosis and conjunctival injection may be seen. These children may or may not have signs suggestive of sinus infection such as malodorous breath, tenderness to palpation, postnasal drip or chronic nocturnal cough. In many cases, a CAT scan of the orbit is necessary in making the correct diagnosis.

A 3-year-old boy fell 4 feet from a sliding board ladder onto concrete. His mother witnessed the fall. For a second he was stunned but then began shrieking. After comforting for several minutes, they walked home together and ate lunch. He napped at his usual time. His mother went to awaken him after 2 hours, thinking that it was unusual for him to sleep so long. He was difficult to arouse, but did open his eyes. She called 911 and the child was brought to the emergency department. On arrival, he is comatose with a Glasgow Coma Score of 6. His left pupil is 5 mm in diameter and his right pupil is 3 mm; both are responsive to light. You find no focal abnormalities on neurologic examination.

1. The first thing you do is:
   A. Give dexamethasone
   B. Proceed to the arteriography suite
   C. Give mannitol
   D. Intubate and hyperventilate
   E. Drill a burr hole

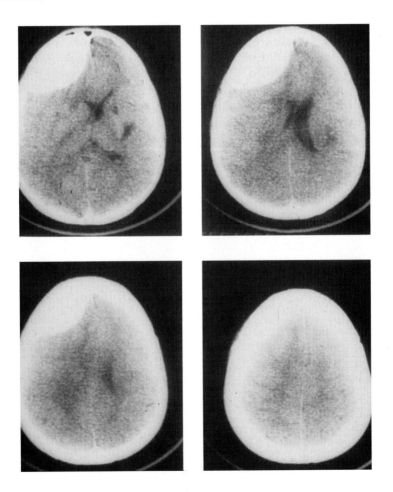

DISCUSSION

ANSWER:

1. **D. Intubate and hyperventilate**

1. Upon arrival to the emergency department, this child has physical examination findings consistent with elevated intracranial pressure and early herniation following blunt head trauma. In the image provided, the typical crescentic density representing epidural blood is present. There is also compression of the lateral ventricle with midline shift, documenting elevated intracranial pressure. Immediate endotracheal intubation and mild hyperventilation to maintain a pCO2 of 30-35 mm Hg will reduce cerebral blood flow (while maintaining adequate perfusion) and may be life saving. Osmolar therapy may provide some benefit in acutely decreasing intracranial pressure; however, it should not precede management with hyperventilation. Further cranial imaging is unnecessary, and dexamethasone is not recommended acutely for the treatment of increased intracranial pressure. Although this patient needs a burr hole, it would be best performed by a neurosurgeon in the operating room.

Further Discussion

Collection of epidural blood results from disruption of arteries or veins in the space between the dura and the calvarium. In children, bleeding often occurs without a skull fracture. The classic presentation of patients with an epidural hematoma includes a history of head trauma with brief altered consciousness followed by a lucid interval then lethargy progressing to coma. In actuality, one-third of patients will have these findings, one-third never lose consciousness, and one-third have altered mental status from the time of the injury. The typical physical findings in addition to coma include dilation of the ipsilateral pupil and contralateral hemiparesis due to compression of the third nerve and the cerebral peduncle as herniation occurs. Immediate recognition and treatment of this clinical entity is important in attempting to reduce permanent brain injury. In some patients, there is no underlying parenchymal injury, and full recovery may occur.

The mother of a 6-month-old child brings her to the emergency department for a problem with her colostomy.

1. The next step is:
   A. Contrast enema
   B. Surgical repair
   C. Intravenous antibiotics
   D. Manual reduction
   E. Narcotic administration

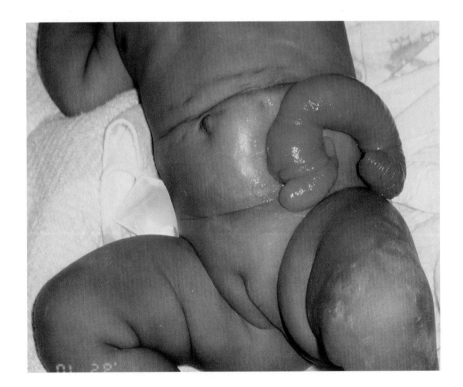

DISCUSSION

ANSWER:

1. D. Manual reduction

1. The bowel has herniated through this infant's colostomy and needs to be reduced promptly. Although sedation with narcotics may help with reduction, this measure is usually unnecessary and not the next step, until an initial attempt has been made. The longer the bowel is prolapsed, the greater the edema, thereby lessening the likelihood of a successful reduction. Failure to achieve a reduction should lead to operative intervention in short order. Further definition of the anatomy with a contrast enema or other imaging study will waste time and contribute nothing. Antibiotics are not a priority unless the patient manifests signs of sepsis.

Further Discussion

Prolapsed bowel through a colostomy is somewhat unusual, as compared to a prolapsed rectum, which is seen frequently in children. Rectal prolapse most often occurs due to an underlying disorder that leads to prolonged coughing, straining at stooling, or neuromuscular impairment; examples include cystic fibrosis, celiac disease, rectal polyps, constipation, chronic diarrhea, ascites, and meningomyelocele. Reduction of a rectal prolapse is achieved with gentle bimanual pressure.

A 3-year-old girl is transferred from another hospital for evaluation of a cervical spine injury. She was hit by a slow-moving vehicle and pushed to the ground. There was no loss of consciousness and she has had a normal mental status since the accident. She has no tenderness in her neck, and her neurologic examination is normal.

1. The appropriate next step is:
   A. Flexion and extension X-rays of the cervical spine
   B. CT scan of the cervical spine
   C. MRI of the cervical spine
   D. Orthopedic consultation
   E. None of the above

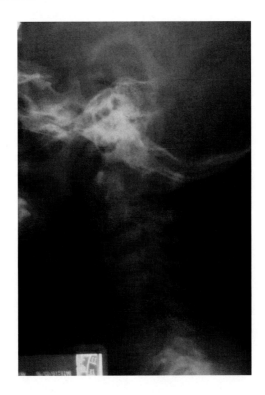

DISCUSSION

ANSWER:

1. **E. None of the above**

1. No further studies are needed. In the X-ray, anterior displacement of the body of C2 on C3 is clearly seen. There are no other abnormalities appreciated. When the posterior cervical line is applied, the diagnosis of physiologic subluxation or pseudo-subluxation is made. Extension and flexion views are sometimes used to accentuate subluxation when it is present. Although obtained unnecessarily here, note that the flexion and extension views (X-rays below) confirm the absence of subluxation. Similarly, both CT and MRI would be non-revealing. This 3-year-old child had a normal physical examination and experienced a low impact injury. After review of the history, physical examination and the radiographs, her cervical collar was removed and she was sent home.

Further Discussion

As with the other bones of the skeleton, the pediatric cervical spine has some unique characteristics. Children have more horizontal facet joints and greater ligamentous laxity than adults. The head is relatively larger, placing the fulcrum of the cervical spine at C2-C3 rather than C5-C6-C7 as it is in the adult spine. Additionally, different age groups have different degrees of ossification, making radiograph interpretation more challenging.

Pseudosubluxation is often noted in young children because of the anatomic features described above. It is seen at C2-C3 or C3-C4, when the neck is in the flexed position. Radiologists often employ the posterior cervical line, or Swischuk's line, to determine whether or not true subluxation exists. This involves drawing a line from the anterior cortex of the spinous process of C1 to that of C3. This line should fall within 2 mm of the cortex of the posterior spinous process of C2 under normal conditions. If this is the case, the finding is consistent with physiologic pseudosubluxation. If not, a ligamentous injury is suspected, and the patient should remain immobilized until injury is ruled out using other modalities in addition.

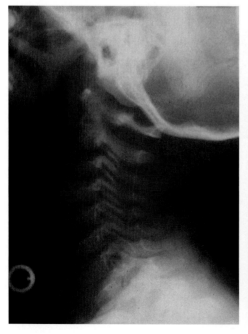
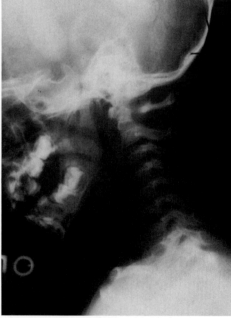

CASE 132

The grandparents of a 5-year-old girl report that she has complained of chest pain intermittently for 2 days. They know she had heart problems but can provide no further details. Her parents are on vacation out of town. On examination, the child appears in no distress. Her vital signs are: P 73/min, R 22/min, BP 105/55 mm Hg, and T 37.3°C. Her neck veins are not distended. An epicardial scar is present. Auscultation reveals a grade II/VI systolic murmur. Her abdomen is nontender without appreciable organomegaly. Femoral pulses are 3+ and symmetric.

The oxygen saturation is 98%.

1. Your immediate therapy is:
    A. Synchronous cardioversion
    B. Transcutaneous pacing
    C. 100% oxygen
    D. Intravenous morphine
    E. None of the above

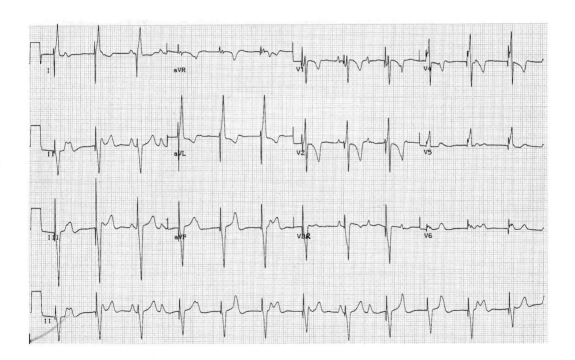

DISCUSSION

ANSWER:

1. E. None of the above

1. This young girl most likely has musculoskeletal chest pain and requires no therapy specifically for her underlying cardiac condition. The EKG shows ventricular pacing at 71 beats per minute, with underlying complete heart block. The findings on this tracing neither account for the chest pain nor call for immediate treatment. While the delivery of 100% oxygen is never wrong, administration is not needed here, given the saturation of nearly 100%. Morphine, used to relieve anginal chest pain in adults, also plays an occasional role in pediatrics among children with "tet" spells, which are characterized by the sudden onset of cyanosis with uncorrected Tetralogy of Fallot and structurally related lesions. Synchronous cardioversion would be indicated for selected patients with either ventricular or supraventricular tachycardias. Transcutaneous pacing may be effective in children with symptomatic bradyarrhythmia with a malfunctioning permanent pacemaker, but has no place in this case.

Further Discussion

With the dramatic advances made by pediatric cardiologists and cardiac surgeons, increasing numbers of children are surviving with arrhythmias after repair of complex congenital heart diseases. Sorting out the correct approach often requires consultation with a cardiologist, especially when an implanted pacemaker needs to be reset or fails to function properly. Fortunately, many of the complaints in these children turn out to be unrelated to the cardiac pathology, as in this case.

An 11-year-old girl comes to the emergency department with a 1 week history of cough. She has had some congestion and low-grade fever for several weeks, and her mother thinks she has lost some weight since moving to the United States 6 months ago. The child has not had any prior medical problems, and she has never been treated for reactive airway disease, although there is a strong family history of atopy. On physical examination, her temperature is 38°C, her respiratory rate is 22/min, and her heart rate is 90/min. She is well-appearing, but coughs frequently during the examination. Her HEENT exam is normal, and her breath sounds are equal bilaterally, with some scattered rhonchi. You decide to give her inhalation beta-agonist therapy while she awaits her chest radiograph.

1. The most appropriate therapy for this child is likely to include:
   A. Prednisone
   B. Vincristine
   C. Amphotericin
   D. Rifampin
   E. Zoduvidine

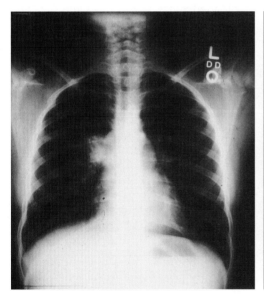
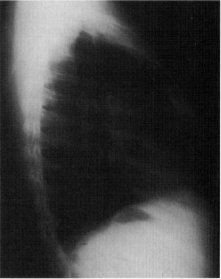

DISCUSSION

ANSWER:

1. D. Rifampin

1. Unilateral hilar adenopathy, as seen on the X-ray, is a hallmark of primary pulmonary tuberculosis, that requires treatment with rifampin and several other anti-tuberculous agents. Some of the other diseases causing hilar adenopathy include lymphoma, HIV, histoplasmosis, and sarcoidosis. Generally, these disorders occur less frequently than tuberculosis and are more likely to cause bilaterally enlarged lymph nodes. Prednisone has a role in several of these diseases, including sarcoidosis and lymphoma. Vincristine is one of the chemotherapeutic agents use for children with lymphoma, amphotericin treats histoplasmosis and other systemic fungal infections, and zoduvidine is a mainstay of therapy in pediatric AIDS.

Further Discussion

Hilar adenopathy can be difficult to diagnosis with certainty on standard radiographs, and often, further imaging of the chest (with a CT scan, for example) is required for assessing the hilar region. Careful review of the lateral chest film avoids mistaking the adenopathy for a perihilar pneumonia. On the lateral view, the vessels in the hilar area normally form a horseshoe density. When hilar adenopathy is present, the density of subcarinal nodes converts this horseshoe into a doughnut.

In addition to hilar adenopathy, several features in the history point to the possibility of tuberculosis. These include birth outside the United States, weight loss, and the chronicity of the fever. Not unexpectedly, the physical examination offers no specific findings.

In over 95% of tuberculosis cases in children, the lung is the initial site of infection. The primary pulmonary complex consists of a focus of tubercle bacilli with surrounding inflammation, lymphangitis and adenitis. Right hilar adenopathy is nicely demonstrated on this child's chest X-ray. This adenopathy in association with bronchial inflammation may lead to obstructive emphysema or segmental atelectasis.

CASE 134

A 13-month-old is brought by her aunt, who reports that the parents dropped the child off at 8:00 a.m. for "baby sitting." As the morning progressed, the child became fussy and refused to walk. When the aunt removed the child's clothes, she noted a "rash."

Vital signs: P 110/min   R 24/min   BP 110/65 mm Hg   T 37.8°C
HEENT   No pharyngeal inflammation
Neck   Minimal shoddy anterior cervical adenopathy
Lungs   Clear to auscultation
Heart   No murmur
Abdomen   No hepatosplenomegaly

1. Your initial diagnostic impression is:
   A. Acute lymphocytic leukemia
   B. Meningococcemia
   C. Trauma (child abuse)
   D. Idiopathic thrombocytopenic
      purpura
   E. Henoch Schönlein purpura

2. The laboratory test most likely to be
   helpful is:
   A. Bone marrow aspiration
   B. Complete blood count
   C. Blood culture
   D. Prothrombin time
   E. Skin biopsy

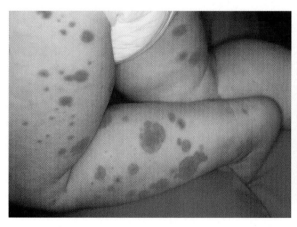
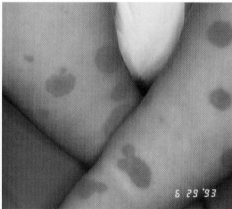

DISCUSSION

ANSWERS:
1. E. Henoch Schonlein purpura
2. B. Complete blood count

1. The appearance of the rash suggests Henoch Schönlein purpura (HSP). Bruising due to meningococcemia is possible, but with this many purpura one would expect a child with bacterial sepsis to be very toxic-appearing and in a state of cardiovascular collapse. Child abuse may result in multiple bruises, but this would be an extraordinary number. Additionally, it would be unlikely that the abused child would have contusions that all appeared round and in the same stage of evolution. With acute lymphoblastic leukemia (ALL), one would expect a more gradual onset and other findings, such as fever, lymphadenopathy, and hepatosplenomegaly. Idiopathic thrombocytopenic purpura (ITP) is characterized by a predominance of petechiae in a generalized distribution, rather than by purpura clustered on the lower extremities.

2. While there is no study that is diagnostic in HSP, a complete blood count (CBC) is indicated to exclude or rule against some of the more serious diseases that enter into the differential diagnosis, including leukemia, sepsis, and ITP. Bone marrow aspiration is performed to confirm leukemia and is often done in cases of ITP, particularly when corticosteroids will be administered for therapy. If this child was febrile, a blood culture for *Neisseria meningitidis* and other pathogens would be appropriate. Clotting studies are useful to diagnose a coagulopathy, either congenital or acquired. In general, skin biopsy is reserved for persistent eruptions that cannot be diagnosed with studies of the blood and consultation.

Further Discussion

HSP is thought to be triggered by minor infections with viruses or bacteria, particularly streptococci. Although the patients are generally well-appearing, some may be fussy due to swelling of the joints. Individual lesions appear to be bruises at first glance but often have an urticarial quality to them as well. The distribution in the dependent areas of buttocks and lower extremities is classic, but lesions may occur on the upper body and arms. Beyond the clinical features, the most important test is the CBC. The finding of normal-appearing white blood cells and a normal platelet count rules out two other important diagnoses, ITP and ALL.

The parents of a 10-year-old girl are concerned that her neck appears swollen. The child has complained of a minor sore throat and has had a tactile fever. On examination, her temperature is 38.6°C and she has erythematous, moderately enlarged tonsils with whitish exudate. Her spleen tip is palpable just below the rib border on the left.

1. The best approach to confirm the diagnosis is:
   A. Complete blood count
   B. Heterophil titer
   C. Aspiration and culture
   D. Rubella antibodies
   E. Tine test

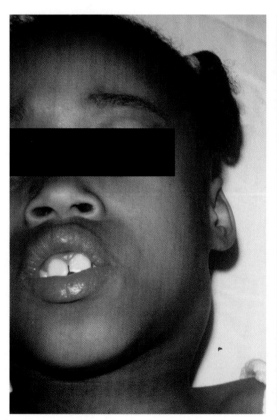
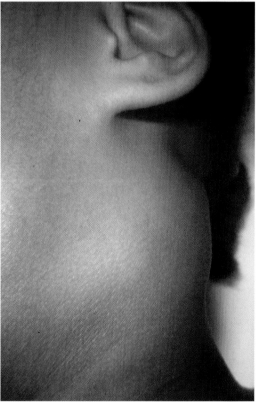

DISCUSSION

ANSWER:

1. **B. Heterophil titer**

1. The finding of a large cluster of nodes, in both the anterior and more particularly the posterior cervical regions, without signs of bacterial adenitis (redness, warmth, tenderness) leads to the diagnosis of infectious mononucleosis. Given the age (>5 years) and the presence of a characteristic infectious mononucleosis syndrome (fever, pharyngitis, adenopathy, and splenomegaly), the heterophil antibody titer (Monospot®) would be the best diagnostic tool. Hints to the diagnosis are the exudative tonsillitis and an enlarged spleen. A complete blood count would almost certainly show atypical lymphocytosis, but this result is less specific than the heterophil titer. The absence of a single, red, fluctuant node points away from a bacterial lymphadenitis, for which aspiration and culture are an excellent approach. Rubella does produce posterior cervical node enlargement, but generally not to this extent. Additionally, one would expect a viral prodrome, a maculopapular rash, and no palpable spleen. Tuberculous adenitis is rare in the United States and usually occurs as a complication of a pulmonary focus.

Further Discussion

Infectious mononucleosis, caused by infection with the Epstein Barr virus, causes many different clinical pictures, from a subclinical infection in the young, through a mild but persistent pharyngitis, to a debilitating illness in the high school aged student, lasting from weeks to months. Posterior cervical adenopathy, as shown here, is the most characteristic feature of the illness. Although a variety of pathogens, particularly the Group A streptococci, may cause marked anterior cervical lymph node enlargement, infection with these organisms does not involve the posterior cervical region. For the majority of patients, diagnosis relies on the detection of heterophil antibodies, most frequently using commercial "spot" kits. Children under 5 years old are less likely than older patients to have a detectable heterophil antibody titer, but it is still worthwhile to run the test, as some manifest a typical response.

A 14-year-old female comes to the emergency department with palpitations. Her history includes a Fontan procedure for tricuspid atresia. Her vital signs are stable and her cardiac rhythm is irregular.

1. Initial therapy would consist of:
    A. Cardioversion
    B. Adenosine
    C. Procainamide
    D. Quinidine
    E. Digoxin

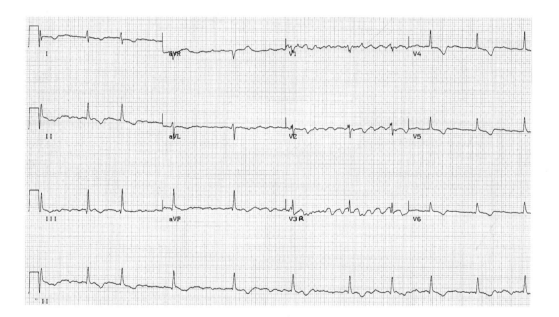

DISCUSSION

ANSWER:

1. E. Digoxin

1. The tracing shows atrial fibrillation with an irregular ventricular response, ranging from 50 to 80 beats per minute. P waves are not seen. The atrial waves are irregular and best seen in leads V1 and V2. There is inferolateral T wave inversion. Since the patient is stable, immediate cardioversion would not be indicated. Adenosine would transiently increase the AV block and might help confirm the diagnosis, but would not be therapeutic. The most commonly recommended initial therapy is digoxin, especially if the ventricular response is fast. When a patient is tachycardic, digoxin slows the ventricular rate, although the atrial fibrillation may persist. Digoxin is often initiated after hospitalization and should not be used if the patient has Wolff-Parkinson-White syndrome. When use of digoxin is unsuccessful after 24 hours, procainamide or quinidine is often tried, but these drugs are not used initially.

Further Discussion

Atrial fibrillation is rare in children and usually occurs in association with either structural heart disease, such as mitral valve disease (resulting in stretched atria), or after surgery involving the atrium, as in this patient. Even more rarely, atrial fibrillation may be seen in a previously normal heart associated with pericarditis, hyperthyroidism, or pulmonary embolism.

The Fontan procedure is the definitive repair for tricuspid atresia and all forms of single ventricle. The systemic venous return is directed to the pulmonary system, bypassing the right ventricle. Connections may vary, but they usually involve either attaching the right atrium directly to the main pulmonary artery or attaching the superior vena cava (SVC) return directly to the right pulmonary artery and attaching the inferior vena cava (IVC) return through an intra-atrial graft to the SVC. Late complications of this life-preserving procedure include supraventricular dysrhythmias (such as atrial fibrillation, atrial flutter, and paroxysmal atrial tachycardia), obstruction to SVC flow causing SVC syndrome, and sudden death.

A 5-week-old infant has a 1-day history of lethargy, fever, vomiting and explosive diarrhea. On physical examination, he is ill-appearing, febrile, and tachycardic with abdominal distension and cool distal extremities. He was a full-term infant and is bottle fed. He has had problems with constipation since birth, which have responded to glycerin suppositories.

1. The most reliable test for making the diagnosis of this condition is:
   A. Abdominal ultrasound
   B. Upper GI
   C. Colonoscopy
   D. Rectal biopsy
   E. Barium enema

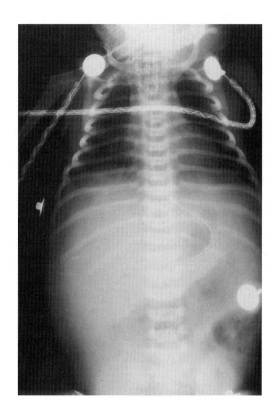

DISCUSSION

ANSWER:

D. Rectal biopsy

1. The infant has Hirschsprung's disease, diagnosed most reliably by rectal biopsy or rectal manometry. Although a barium enema may be strongly suggestive, it is often negative in young infants. Abdominal ultrasound at this age is an excellent modality for imaging pyloric stenosis and helpful in some cases of intussusception and volvulus. An upper gastrointestinal series is useful for identifying malrotation of the intestines. Colonoscopy is rarely, if ever, indicated in the initial evaluation of an infant with an acute obstruction.

Further Discussion

This young infant presented with symptoms consistent with enterocolitis, that occurred as a complication of Hirschsprung's disease. The diagnosis in this child was made during exploratory laparotomy. On viewing the abdominal X-ray, distended loops of bowel are noted. There is no clear evidence of mechanical obstruction and no free air or pneumatosis. This infant's history includes constipation and feeding intolerance since birth, and he now presents with shock, abdominal distension and diarrhea. If not recognized promptly, enterocolitis has a significant morbidity and mortality. Immediate fluid resuscitation is necessary to improve oxygen delivery to all the vital organs. Antibiotic therapy for suspected abdominal catastrophes should include coverage of intestinal flora. Cefoxitin or a combination of ampicillin, gentamicin and clindamycin are reasonable choices.

In Hirschsprung's disease, there is an absence of ganglionic cells between the circular and longitudinal muscle layers of the bowel that results in abnormal intestinal motility. The area of the rectosigmoid is the most common segment of bowel involved. The clinical signs of this disease are highly variable and may go undiagnosed into adulthood. Newborns may present in the first days of life with abdominal distention, vomiting and failure to pass meconium, or they may develop only constipation early on and then present later with severe obstruction or enterocolitis. Delayed passage of meconium is present in over 90% of patients in whom this diagnosis is made. In the older infant and child, there is almost always a history of waxing and waning constipation. On physical examination in the classic example, no stool is appreciated in the rectal vault, in marked contrast to the usual finding in patients with functional constipation. A dilated transverse colon along with fecal impaction may be palpable during examination of the abdomen.

A barium enema may be normal or, as shown in the X-ray on the followng page, may reveal a narrow segment with dilated proximal bowel, that is consistent with Hirschprung's disease. Dilation of the proximal bowel may be absent, particularly during the first months of life. An X-ray taken after 24 hours showing retained barium at the transition zone aids in making the diagnosis. Anorectal manometry and rectal biopsy may be necessary for confirmation.

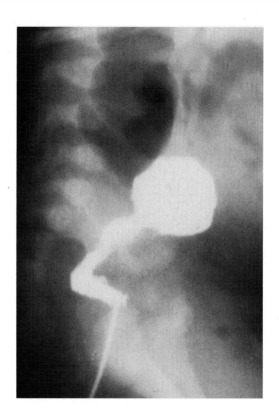

This 9-year-old boy presents with a pruritic rash for 24 hours. Yesterday his mother noted two lesions on his back, which appeared after she had been playing with the family dog, but today he has at least 50 lesions. His temperature is 38°C.

1. What is the most likely cause of this rash?
   A. Flea bites
   B. Rickettsial pox
   C. Mucha-Habermann disease
   D. Dermatitis herpetiformis
   E. Varicella

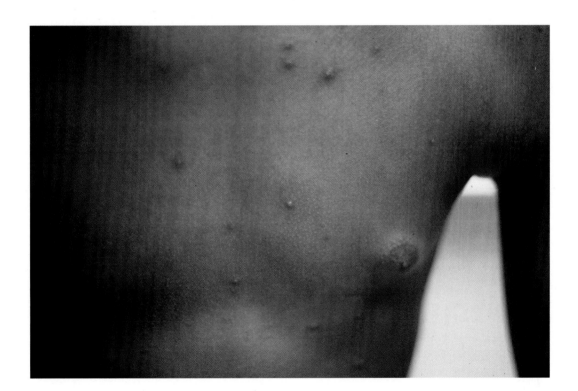

DISCUSSION

ANSWER:

1. E. Varicella

1. Sorry, no zebras here, this patient has varicella (chickenpox). Although some constitutional symptoms may precede the rash, the patients usually seek care only when the rash appears. A rapid onset as in this case is common, with a few lesions noted one afternoon and full-blown varicella the next day. The rash begins centrally on the trunk and face as tiny macules, then papules, then clear 1-2 mm vesicles on an erythematous base, progressing to crusting over 24 to 48 hours. Different stages of the rash may coexist in time and location. The mucous membranes are usually also involved (e.g., mouth, palate, tonsils, conjunctiva, and vagina). Patients are frequently febrile for the first few days of the illness.

Flea bites can be easily mistaken for varicella, when they appear as small, pruritic vesicles. With flea bites, there are usually fewer lesions than with varicella, constitutional symptoms are lacking, and the vesicles sit on a larger, erythematous swollen area. The red area associated with flea bites is usually 1-3 cm across compared to just a few millimeters of erythema surrounding a noninfected varicella lesion.

Rickettsial pox is occasionally seen in urban areas of the eastern United States. It is caused by *Rickettsia akari* transmitted from mites to humans. Unlike varicella where the patient is only mildly ill for a day prior to the rash, in rickettsial pox the patient is usually ill for a week with high fever, chills, myalgias and headache. The rash consists of erythematous maculopapular lesions that later develop a vesicle mounted on the preexisting lesions.

Mucha-Habermann disease, also known as pityriasis lichenoides et varioliformis acuta (PLEVA), has no known etiology and rarely has constitutional symptoms. The rash begins as red maculas and papules but soon evolves into vesicles that necrose and become purpuric. Although the trunk is involved as with varicella, the rash is most pronounced on the flexor surfaces of the extremities while the face and mucous membranes are spared. The lesions last for weeks or even months. Consider PLEVA if you see a rash that is similar to but not completely typical for varicella and does not resolve.

Dermatitis herpetiformis is a recurrent blistering disease of children over 8 years of age. The vesicles are 1-4 mm, extremely pruritic, and appear in groups over extensor surfaces (e.g., elbows, knees, shoulders or buttocks). Mucous membranes are spared. Cutaneous biopsy is frequently needed to confirm the diagnosis.

Further Discussion

Despite licensure of a vaccine for varicella, many cases and complications continue to occur. Beware of the child who has high fevers after the fifth day of the rash or extremity pain or swelling, as these symptoms suggest possible streptococcal superinfection.

The father of a 4-year-old girl complains that she has had increasing fatigue, a "weak" neck, and a "droopy eye" for several days. He has not observed her to have fever, headache, vomiting, and limp. This morning before leaving for work, he thought the illness had resolved, but he became alarmed by "how bad" she looked when he returned from the office at dinnertime. Her temperature is 36.8°C. The examination is normal except as shown.

1. What study would you recommend?
   A. Lumbar puncture
   B. T_4 and TSH levels
   C. Electromyography
   D. Head CT scan
   E. Edrophonium infusion

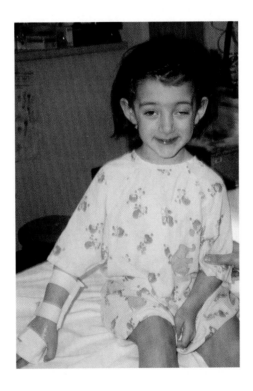

DISCUSSION

ANSWER:

1. E. Edrophonium infusion

1. The photograph shows an alert child with left sided ptosis. Although a patient can appear to have ptosis due to lid inflammation, infection, or trauma, this child's lid is not swollen or red. The cause of the ptosis in this case is myasthenia gravis, which is diagnosed by the response to edrophonium (Tensilon®) infusion. Myasthenia gravis is suggested by the finding of isolated ptosis in an otherwise well-appearing child, particularly with a history of deterioration late in the day. Hyperthyroidism, confirmed by measurement of T_4 and TSH levels, is associated with ophthalmoplegia, and patients may have lid lag on downward gaze, but do not usually have ptosis. Infantile botulism causes decreased activity and constipation, and examination may reveal hypotonia and ptosis. The diagnosis is confirmed by electromyography. This child is too old for the infantile form. Intracranial masses causing increased intracranial pressure may present with headache, vomiting, and isolated cranial nerve palsies, most commonly involving the lateral rectus muscle. A head CT is the best initial imaging modality.

Further Discussion

The symptoms of myasthenia gravis are caused by an immune mediated neuromuscular blockade. Acetylcholine receptor antibodies bind receptors on the motor end plate, decreasing available sites for the physiologic acetylcholine-mediated motor end plate response. This results in the rapid fatigue of muscles. For example, this patient's ptosis will increase if she tries to prolong her upward gaze for 1 to 2 minutes. Ophthalmoplegia, facial weakness, dysphagia, neck or extremity weakness may all occur. Tensilon® (edrophonium chloride) is a cholinesterase inhibitor, inhibiting acetylcholine hydrolysis and thereby prolonging the effects of acetylcholine. This reverses the signs of myasthenia for a few minutes. Resuscitation equipment and atropine should be available when infusing edrophonium, as isolated cases of respiratory arrest have been reported. The initial dose of edrophonium should be .02 mg per kg IV (1/10th the full dose). If tolerated, administer the full dose of 0.2 mg per kg (maximum dose 10 mg). Deliver 1/5th the dose over 1 minute and if no response in 45 seconds, give the remainder.

This child's response to Tensilon is shown in the following photograph.

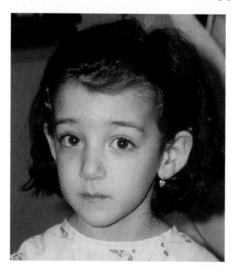

This previously healthy 3-year-old girl has had a presumed upper respiratory infection for the past 4 days. On the morning of this visit, the child vomited three times and the mother felt the child was "just not acting herself." Her temperature is 39.8°C.

1. The procedure most likely to provide a diagnosis is a:
   A. CT scan of the head
   B. Lumbar puncture
   C. Fluorescein stain
   D. Cervical spine X-ray
   E. Otoscopic examination

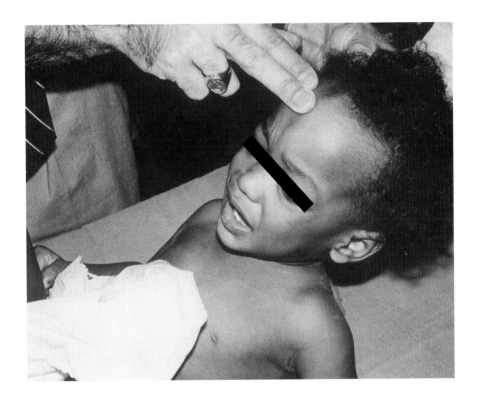

DISCUSSION

ANSWER:

1. **B. Lumbar puncture**

1. As her neck is flexed, this girl grimaces and brings her shoulders up off the stretcher, demonstrating nuchal rigidity. Moments later, a lumbar puncture demonstrated purulent spinal fluid from bacterial meningitis. Vertebral osteomyelitis, which may cause neck pain and nuchal rigidity, is best diagnosed by bone scan or MRI, but may produce abnormalities on cervical spine X-rays. Mass lesions may present with lethargy and neck stiffness, but represent a relatively uncommon etiology in previously healthy, febrile patients who become ill acutely; CT scans are generally quite useful for diagnosing tumors. Both otitis media and corneal abrasion are explanations for irritability, but not for nuchal rigidity.

Further Discussion

Nuchal rigidity, one of the classic signs of meningitis, is rare in the first few months of life, unreliable before one year of age, and occasionally absent in older children and adults. The finding of nuchal rigidity in a febrile child suggests meningitis, but is not conclusive. Other causes of neck stiffness include trauma, myositis, adenitis, retropharyngeal abscess, and upper lobe pneumonia.

The introduction of conjugated vaccines against *Hemophilus influenzae* has reduced dramatically the incidence of meningitis in childhood. Yet both *Streptococcus pneumoniae* and *Neisseria meningitidis* infect the central nervous system of thousands of children each year. Continued vigilance is warranted.

A 10-year-old girl fell over the banister at school from the second to the first floor. She landed on her left shoulder and had no loss of consciousness at the scene. She was immobilized by the paramedics and brought to the emergency department. On arrival she is awake and alert. Her pulse is 130/min, her respiratory rate is 30/min, and her blood pressure is 110/70 mm Hg.

1. What injury do you suspect?
    A. Liver laceration
    B. Splenic laceration
    C. Renal contusion
    D. Duodenal hematoma
    E. Bowel rupture

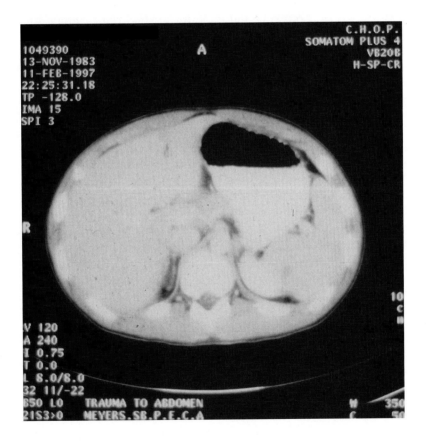

DISCUSSION

ANSWER:

1. B. Splenic laceration

1. Considering the mechanism of injury and evidence of intravascular depletion, an occult abdominal injury is highly likely. The abdominal CT scan of this child shows the presence of a splenic laceration. The spleen and the liver are the abdominal organs most commonly injured in children. The majority of these injuries occur following motor vehicle accidents. Falls, sports injuries and direct blows to the area are also important mechanisms of injury. Children may complain of left abdominal or flank discomfort, or pain may be referred to the shoulder (Kehr's sign). They may have shortness of breath, nausea or vomiting. Physical signs are present in only 60% of patients and may include tachypnea, tachycardia, hypotension, abdominal tenderness or abdominal/flank ecchymosis.

Further Discussion

Currently, the abdominal CT scan is the study of choice in most pediatric centers for evaluating injured children. It is fast and sensitive in detecting intra- and/or retroperitoneal fluid or blood, as well as identifying and quantifying solid organ injury. Injuries to the bowel and pancreas may be missed, but are not common. Indications for performing the study include severe mechanism of injury, symptoms or signs suggestive of an abdominal injury, evidence of multisystem trauma, head injury with a decreased level of consciousness, and asymptomatic gross hematuria. Diagnostic peritoneal lavage (DPL) may miss retroperitoneal blood and small subcapsular liver or spleen hematomas, and may lead to unnecessary laparotomy. Ultrasound as the initial imaging modality is still under evaluation.

Over the past decade, selective non-operative management of blunt abdominal trauma resulting in injury to the solid abdominal organs has become the treatment of choice. If hemodynamically stable, most children with blunt abdominal injury may be followed nonoperatively. Hospital bed rest and observation are recommended for 5 to 7 days, although some surgeons allow a shorter period. Activities are restricted for 8 weeks following discharge. Non-operative management in selected patients with injuries to the spleen has greatly reduced the morbidity and mortality associated with splenectomy and its increased risk of infection with encapsulated organisms.

This 7-year-old girl with leukemia was seen 3 days ago for a rash that has progressed. Currently, she appears acutely ill and is febrile to 39°C.

1. Upon her initial presentation, the most appropriate treatment would have been:
   A. VZIG
   B. Amphotericin
   C. Acyclovir
   D. Ceftriaxone
   E. Fresh frozen plasma

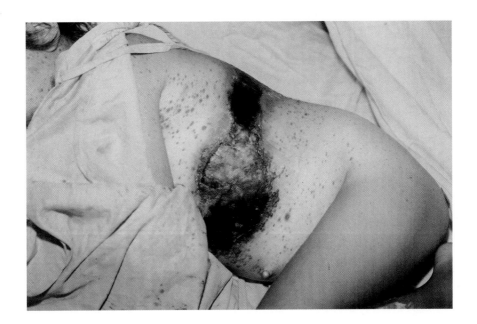

DISCUSSION

ANSWER:

1. C. Acyclovir

1. This youngster with leukemia has a severe eruption of herpes zoster, which eventually proved fatal. When an immunosuppressed child develops either varicella or zoster, intravenous acyclovir therapy is recommended. VZIG plays a role in exposures, but not for established infections. Neither antibacterial (ceftriaxone) nor antifungal therapy (amphotericin) will help in this situation unless secondary infection develops. Fresh frozen plasma is not useful either for prophylaxis or therapy.

Further Discussion

Although severe infections such as the one in this case are rare, both exposures (varicella) and initial mild eruptions (varicella or zoster) are common. It is important to carefully assess these situations to prevent complications. Untreated varicella or zoster in the immunosuppressed host has a mortality rate in the range of 10%. If a susceptible patient reports an exposure within 72 hours, VZIG should be administered in a dose of 0.2 vials/kg. Once the rash occurs, intravenous acyclovir is the treatment of choice. When uncertain about the etiology of a vesicular rash, either perform a rapid immunofluorescence study on a scraping of the lesion or err on the side of therapy.

An 11-year-old boy is transported to the emergency department after he was hit by a stray bullet. He is cardiovascularly stable and the primary survey reveals no acutely life-threatening injuries. An entry wound is seen on his medial thigh. His vital signs are as follows: P 110/min; R 18/min; BP 115/80 mm Hg.

1. Given that he is stable, your most important task is to determine if he has:
   A. Skeletal injuries
   B. Peripheral nerve injuries
   C. Intra-abdominal injuries
   D. Peripheral vascular injuries
   E. Compartment syndrome.

2. If he develops a diminished peripheral pulse in the extremity or an expanding pulsatile hematoma, your next step should be:
   A. Plain radiographs of the femur
   B. Arteriography
   C. Doppler ultrasound
   D. Surgical consultation
   E. Admission and observation

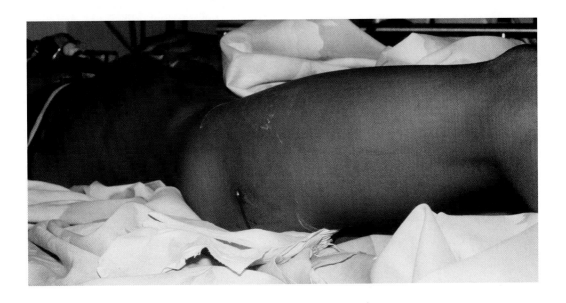

DISCUSSION

ANSWERS:

1. C. Intra-abdominal injuries
2. D. Surgical consultation

1. Although all of these injuries are important, intra-abdominal injuries are most likely to be life-threatening. Not infrequently, a bullet can ricochet off a bone in the proximal portion of an extremity and enter the torso. Next in order of priority would be a vascular injury, which may be limb threatening and is likely to require immediate operation. Skeletal injuries are seen in about 20% of extremity gunshot wounds, and all such injuries should be evaluated radiographically. Peripheral nerve injuries may also occur, especially in association with fractures. Most of these injuries resolve spontaneously and require primary repair only rarely. Compartment syndromes occur more distally, usually in the anterior compartment of the lower leg.

2. Diminished pulses, an expanding pulsatile hematoma, or brisk external bleeding strongly suggest the presence of a vascular injury and a surgeon should be consulted immediately. X-rays are needed, as explained above, but should not delay initiating the consult. Prompt surgical repair to restore blood flow to the extremity within 4 to 6 hours is critical. Arteriography or Doppler ultrasound is not always required if the patient has definitive signs of vascular injury. Admission and observation (with or without further imaging) would be an option, if the patient had only minimal findings, such as a small nonpulsatile hematoma.

Further Discussion

Arteriography has been the gold standard for identifying vascular injury that requires surgical exploration. When used by an experienced operator, Doppler ultrasound detects 60-80% of arterial injuries, and the missed injuries usually do not require surgical repair. Some experts suggest that physical examination and 24 hours of observation can also exclude vascular injuries that require surgical repair.

An 8-day-old male is brought to the hospital after "turning blue" at home. In the emergency department, the patient does not appear cyanotic and the vital signs are normal. A grade III/VI harsh systolic ejection murmur is audible at the left upper sternal border. S2 is single. The patient has no hepatosplenomegaly. An EKG is obtained.

1. What might you expect to see on the patient's chest X-ray?
   A. A heart that is large in size and pulmonary venous congestion
   B. A heart that is normal in size and increased pulmonary markings at the bases
   C. A heart that is shaped like a wooden shoe and decreased pulmonary vascular markings
   D. A heart that is shaped like a snowman and increased pulmonary vascular markings
   E. A heart that is normal in size and normal pulmonary vascular markings

2. When the patient returns from radiology, you are called to the room. The infant is crying, tachypneic and extremely cyanotic. What should you do immediately?
   A. Obtain an arterial blood gas
   B. Intubate the child
   C. Administer subcutaneous morphine
   D. Give intravenous furosemide
   E. Arrange for immediate catheterization

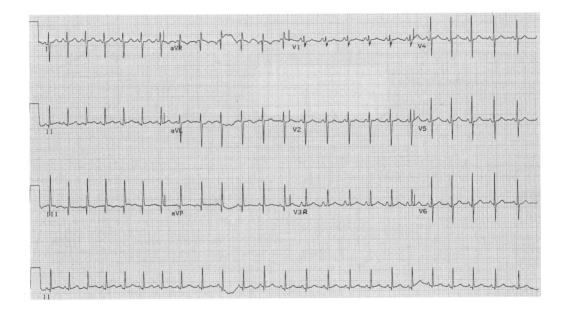

DISCUSSION

ANSWERS:

1. C. A heart that is shaped like a wooden shoe and decreased pulmonary vascular markings
2. C. Administer subcutaneous morphine

1. The EKG shows sinus rhythm, a rightward axis (normal for age), and right ventricular hypertrophy indicated by a tall R wave in V3R, a deep S wave in lead V6, and an upright T wave in leads V3R and V1. Remember that after about 3 days of age the T wave is inverted in lead V1 and only becomes upright in adolescence. The history of a cyanotic spell, the cardiac examination consistent with pulmonary stenosis, and an EKG with right ventricular hypertrophy are suggestive of Tetralogy of Fallot. This congenital defect usually consists of pulmonary stenosis, a ventricular septal defect, and an aorta that overrides the ventricular septum. The X-ray in a patient with Tetralogy of Fallot shows a heart with a characteristic appearance. The heart size is normal and the pulmonary vascular markings are decreased due to the severe pulmonary stenosis. The elevated apex (resembling a wooden shoe or boot) is due to the right ventricular hypertrophy. In addition, the base of the heart is narrow due to decreased pulmonary artery flow and the overriding aorta that is displaced to the right. Cardiomegaly and pulmonary venous congestion suggest predominant congestive heart failure which might result from coarctation of the aorta or truncus arteriosus. Bilateral diffuse lower lung field infiltrates could be seen if the child had an aspiration pneumonia. A large bilateral supracardiac shadow, with increased pulmonary vascular markings and a snowman appearance are seen with total anomalous pulmonary venous return. Patients with total anomalous pulmonary venous return may have the acute onset of cyanosis and respiratory distress, but often have no murmur at all and do not spontaneously resolve their symptoms; the EKG does demonstrate right axis deviation and right ventricular hypertrophy. Finally, a normal heart size and clear lung fields would be expected in an infant with cyanosis on the basis of neurologic disease.

2. It sounds as if the infant is having a "tet" or "blue spell," seen in patients with Tetralogy of Fallot. These spells often follow episodes of crying and result from an acute decrease in the already compromised pulmonary blood flow. As the patient's right ventricle contracts, unsaturated blood can flow either across the stenotic pulmonary valve into the pulmonary circulation or across the ventricular septal defect (VSD) into the aorta. During the "tet" spell, pulmonary obstruction is acutely increased, possible due to infundibular spasm. This results in more unsaturated blood flowing across the VSD and into the systemic circulation. A spell begins with cyanosis, tachypnea, and restlessness and occasionally progresses to loss of consciousness. The correct therapy for a "tet" spell includes calming the child, positioning to increase pulmonary blood flow (squatting or knee-to-chest position in an older child), and subcutaneous morphine. The morphine acts as a sedative to decrease agitation and tachypnea, which increase oxygen usage. Morphine may also affect pulmonary blood flow. Avoid painful procedures, such as arterial punctures, as a spell begins, since calming the child may abort the episode. Although, in rare cases, a spell may progress and make intubation necessary, reversing the abnormal cardiovascular physiology by positioning and calming the patient and administering morphine should be attempted first. The child has no signs of congestive heart failure, and furosemide is not indicated.

Further Discussion

Cyanotic spells may be due to pulmonary disease, to neurologic illness such as a seizure, to intracranial hemorrhage, to gastrointestinal illness such as gastroesophageal reflux with apnea, to hematological illness such as methemoglobinemia, to cardiac disease, or to apnea from any cause.

A 15-year-old boy complains of neck pain. Yesterday while riding his ten-speed bike he hit a rock and was thrown head first over the handle bars. He denies other injuries. On physical examination, he has tenderness posteriorly over the upper portion of his cervical spine. Range of motion of his neck is limited by pain. A thorough neurologic examination reveals no abnormalities.

1. Upon review of his X-ray, you decide to:
   A. Arrange follow-up with orthopedics
   B. Obtain a CT scan of the neck
   C. Give methylprednisolone
   D. Obtain an MRI of the neck
   E. Discharge him in a soft collar

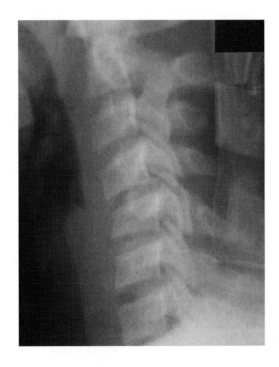

DISCUSSION

ANSWER:

1. **D. Obtain an MRI of the neck**

1. The appropriate decision is to maintain immobilization of the cervical spine, consult a neurosurgeon or orthopedist, and obtain an MRI to better define the injury that you note at C4-C5. A CT scan of the neck is a useful adjunct in identifying bony injury, when an adequate three-view series cannot be obtained. However, the MRI is able to detect and define ligamentous and bony injury, as well as spinal cord injury with greater precision. In this case, given that a subluxation is seen, it makes sense to gain the maximum definition of the injury with MRI. High dose methylprednisolone should be considered if there is evidence on physical examination of neurologic injury or if there is bony injury in a patient with an altered consciousness. Simply arranging follow-up with an orthopedist or discharging the patient in a soft collar is not sufficient.

Further Discussion

Evaluation of the pediatric cervical spine calls for a three-view approach, including lateral, anteroposterior, and open-mouth or odontoid views. The lateral is the most informative view with a sensitivity for identifying injuries of 75-95%. The additional two views increase the sensitivity to greater than 95%. Flexion and extension views are obtained in children complaining of neck pain in whom the three-view series is normal, if ligamentous injury is strongly suspected. These views are also occasionally used to evaluate the magnitude of subluxation.

The lateral X-ray in this case clearly shows anterior subluxation of C4 on C5. There are no bony abnormalities seen. Note that the distance between the interspinous processes of C4 and C5 is widened. On the flexion view below, the abnormalities are striking. Remember that the patient may show minimal to no abnormalities on the neutral lateral view and show considerable abnormalities on the flexion view. An MRI of this boy's neck revealed partial disruption of the posterior longitudinal ligament. He was placed in halo traction but eventually required posterior fusion.

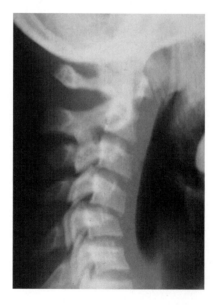

A 10-year-old girl is brought to your emergency department with a painful left hand. She was helping her father plug in an air conditioner about 60 minutes ago, when he heard a loud sound and saw the girl jump away from the outlet. She cried immediately.

1. In addition to what you see in the photograph, the most common physical examination finding you might expect in this patient is:
   A. An irregular pulse
   B. An absent radial pulse
   C. A smaller wound elsewhere
   D. Tonic-clonic activity
   E. Decreasing level of consciousness

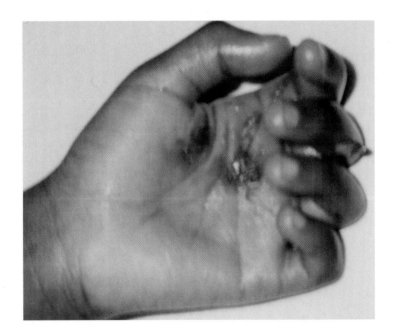

DISCUSSION

ANSWER:

1. **C. A smaller wound elsewhere**

1. Although cardiac dysrhythmias are seen in electrical burns, they usually accompany high voltage injuries (>1,000 volts) or occur when the victim is wet. Water or perspiration decreases skin resistance, allowing increased current flow from the same voltage (Ohm's law). Since this was a low voltage (110- or 220-volt) injury, this child is at a very low risk for cardiac dysrhythmias. Severe electrical burns can cause thrombosis of arteries and absent pulses, but this complication is unlikely in this patient with a superficial injury and obviously well-perfused digits. The most likely finding, although still seen in only a minority of patients, is a smaller wound elsewhere, where the current exits the patient's body to ground. A careful examination of all skin surfaces should be done to look for an exit injury, most commonly involving a foot or the other hand. Frequently the current has only arced across an electrical plug causing a single burn. Although immediate neurological complications, such as loss of consciousness or seizures, may be seen, delayed decreasing level of consciousness or convulsions are rare. Impaired vision or hearing, headaches or amnesia are more common.

Further Discussion

Burn injuries are common, even in low voltage exposures. The injury can be a true electrical burn in which the patient is part of the electrical circuit or a "flash" burn caused by heat from an electrical arc in which the patient is not part of the electrical circuit. In a true electrical burn, the current through the victim causes direct heating of tissue. The extent of the deep tissue damage may be much greater than the skin manifestations and may not be apparent for days. This type of burn can cause myoglobinuria with potential renal failure, or cardiac dysrhythmias. A flash burn is caused by direct thermal injury from an electrical arc outside the patient's body. This child may have had a flash burn if the current jumped across the electrical plug. In a flash burn, no exit wound is seen and complications are limited to those associated with the local thermal injury.

A 7-year-old male is brought to the emergency department with a 2-day history of a painful red eye. He has no history of trauma, and is afebrile. His vision is 20/20.

1. The most likely cause of this patient's illness is:
    A. Allergic reaction
    B. Bacterial infection
    C. Adenoviral infection
    D. Chlamydial infection
    E. Herpetic infection

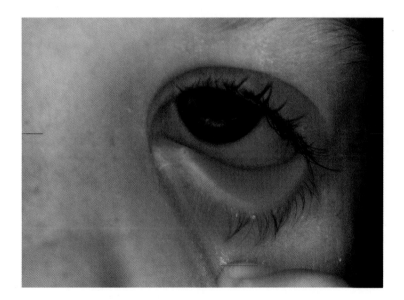

DISCUSSION

ANSWER:

1. C. Adenoviral infection

1. The patient has hemorrhagic bulbar and tarsal conjunctivae. His tarsal conjunctiva does not have any large follicles. Allergic conjunctivitis is more likely to present with an itchy rather than a painful eye, and although the conjunctiva might be injected, it is not hemorrhagic. Bacterial conjunctivitis is not usually painful, and a purulent discharge is prominent. Chlamydial conjunctivitis, caused by an obligate intracellular organism, is transmitted sexually or during passage through the birth canal and more common in adolescents and newborns. The discharge is less purulent than that caused by bacteria, and the conjunctivae are injected but not hemorrhagic. Herpetic conjunctivitis is more common in the neonatal period, and is often associated with skin lesions, clear discharge and injection. Fluorescein staining may show corneal uptake in a dendritic pattern. The most likely cause listed here of this hemorrhagic conjunctivitis is adenoviral, although the specific agent is difficult to predict.

Further Discussion

This patient probably has either epidemic keratoconjunctivitis (EKC), due to adenovirus serotype 8 or 19, or acute hemorrhagic conjunctivitis, usually associated with enterovirus type 70. Both are extremely contagious. EKC presents with an itching or burning sensation, fever, and lid swelling. The conjunctivitis can be hemorrhagic, but frequently the tarsal conjunctiva has large follicles, a preauricular node is swollen, and the patient's vision may be impaired due to corneal involvement. Acute hemorrhagic conjunctivitis presents in a similar fashion and may be associated with seventh cranial nerve paresis.

A 12-year-old girl complains of large "blisters" for several days. She was well until 1 week prior to this visit, when she developed a fever. Four days ago, a rash began on her neck and trunk. New lesions have continued to appear and some have developed into bullae. Her fever has defervesced. On examination, her vital signs are as follows: P 82/min, R 16/min, BP 115/75 mm Hg, and T 37.7°C. Other than the cutaneous finding, her examination is unremarkable.

1. Your diagnosis is:
   A. Varicella
   B. Scalded skin syndrome
   C. Toxic shock syndrome
   D. Epidermolysis bullosa
   E. Toxic epidermonecrolysis

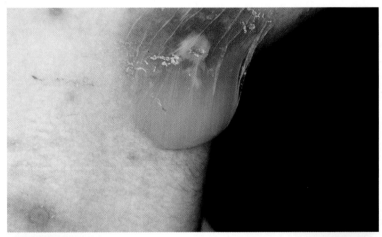

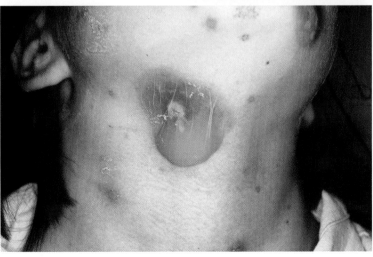

DISCUSSION

ANSWER:

1. A. Varicella

1. This girl has bullous varicella. She has scattered lesions in various stages, including papular, vesicular, bullous, and crusted. While epidermolysis bullosa is characterized by formation of bullae, this disease is a congenital problem rather than an acute illness heralded by fever. Both staphylococcal scalded skin syndrome (SSSS) and toxic epidermolysis (TEN) manifest with areas of desquamation and a positive Nikolsky sign (desquamation of normal skin in response to slight pressure); the former is caused by an infection with *Staphylococcus aureus* and the latter occurs secondary to a drug reaction. Toxic shock syndrome includes fever, hypotension, and a maculopapular rash.

Further Discussion

The most worrisome complications of varicella are encephalitis, Group A streptococcal sepsis, and necrotizing fasciitis. Bullous varicella is far more common, but much less serious, than these. Most commonly a bullous eruption results from secondary staphylococcal infection, but it may also be due simply to a failure to contain the virus; more often seen in immunocompromised hosts, large vesicles or bullae occasionally occur in otherwise healthy patients. The child pictured here was previously well and recovered after treatment with an antistaphylococcal penicillin.

A 5-year-old boy developed a lesion on his wrist approximately 4 days ago. It began as a small red papule and has enlarge gradually. He has not been ill or had any other dermatologic problems. On examination, he appears well and is afebrile.

1. This lesion is best treated by:
   A. Observation
   B. Warm compresses
   C. Incision and drainage
   D. Oral cephalexin
   E. Intravenous oxacillin

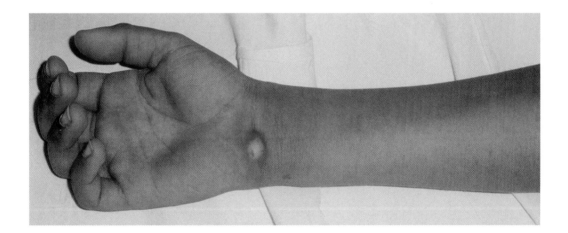

DISCUSSION

ANSWER:

1. C. Incision and drainage

1. The treatment for this superficial abscess is incision and drainage. With observation alone, pus will simply continue to accumulate and the early lymphadenitis that is present will extend. Once a lesion becomes fluctuant, neither compresses nor antibiotics by any route are sufficient to achieve a cure.

Further Discussion

This abscess is located in an area where a number of tendons, a major artery, and two nerves lie just below the surface. Incision and drainage should be performed with great care through a superficial incision. Given the lymphangitis that has developed, the addition of antibiotics to surgical drainage is reasonable, although perhaps more than is necessary. As long as the child is afebrile, oral antibiotics will reliably produce a rapid response.

A 3-year-old boy is transported by ambulance to the emergency department after being struck by a car. He is intubated and being ventilated manually using 100% oxygen, the cervical spine is immobilized, the trachea is midline, breath sounds are equal, pulses are easily palpable, and the extremities are well perfused. His pupils are equal and reactive to light, and he withdraws to painful stimulation. His vital signs are stable, and his oxygen saturation is 100%. The chest X-ray is shown below.

1. After yelling at your colleague about the misplaced nasogastric tube, therapy for this patient should include:
   A. Needle thoracostomy
   B. Chest tube placement
   C. Immediate thoracotomy
   D. Mechanical ventilation
   E. Pericardiocentesis

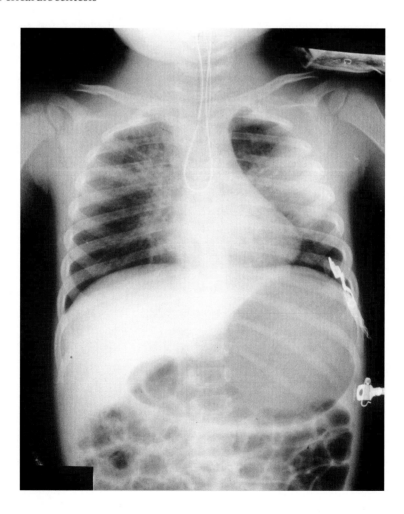

DISCUSSION

ANSWER:

1. **D. Mechanical ventilation**

1. The X-ray shows an area of consolidation of the left mid lung field, probably the lower segment of the left upper lobe. If the child had walked in complaining of fever and cough, this would probably indicate pus in the alveoli, i.e., pneumonia. In the context of trauma, this indicates a pulmonary contusion. A contusion may result in immediate or slowly developing respiratory failure, which may be managed by endotracheal intubation and mechanical ventilation. The only indication for needle thoracostomy is to relieve a tension pneumothorax until a chest tube can be placed. This diagnosis should be suggested clinically, when a patient has respiratory distress, cyanosis, unilaterally decreased breath sounds and possibly tracheal deviation and distended neck veins. A chest tube would be placed for a pneumothorax or large hemothorax. An emergency department thoracotomy should be considered during a traumatic cardiopulmonary arrest, especially for exsanguinating, penetrating precordial injuries. Pericardiocentesis is indicated for cardiac tamponade, usually seen after penetrating trauma, since only a small amount of blood in the pericardial sac can reduce cardiac output. Patients with tamponade usually have muffled heart tones, hypotension or decreased pulse pressure, and distended neck veins. The X-ray may show an enlarged cardiac silhouette. Pericardiocentesis might be considered in any trauma patient whose hypotension does not respond to the usual therapy of hemorrhagic shock.

Further Discussion

Although the mechanism is not known, blunt chest trauma can lead to alveolar edema and hemorrhage, resulting in impaired gas exchange. Symptoms and signs may range from cough and rales to dyspnea, cyanosis and respiratory distress. The X-ray may show an irregular patchy infiltrate or a large consolidation. Remember that the initial contusion may worsen over the next few hours. Therapy depends on symptoms and may range from oxygen and chest physical therapy to endotracheal intubation and bronchial suctioning. Although intravenous fluid overload should be avoided, withholding intravenous fluid will not decrease the alveolar edema and hemorrhage.

The mother of 4-month-old baby wants him evaluated because he seems to bruise easily. During prior visits for well child care, this problem had not been noted. The infant has received all appropriate immunizations without any adverse reactions. The mother, a physician, is adamant about the need for further testing.

1. You suspect the diagnosis is:
   A. Fair skin (normal)
   B. Ehlers Danlos syndrome
   C. Child abuse
   D. Liver disease
   E. Hemophilia

2. Based on your initial impression, you proceed to:
   A. Order a skeletal survey
   B. Arrange a skin biopsy
   C. Draw clotting studies
   D. Send liver enzymes
   E. File a report of abuse

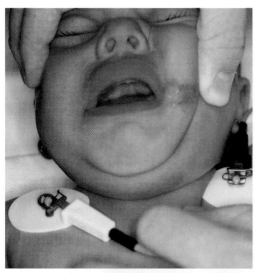
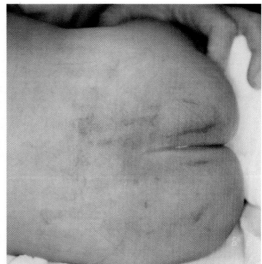
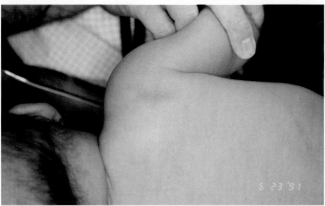

DISCUSSION

ANSWERS:
1. C. Child abuse
2. E. File a report of abuse

1. Any bruise on a young baby must be considered suspicious for child abuse, as in the case in this patient. It is by far the most common diagnosis listed. Ehlers Danlos syndrome is marked by easy bruising and ligamentous laxity. It is a rare condition. Bruises usually occur over areas traumatized by contact with environmental objects, such as the extensor surfaces of the arms and legs. Hemophilia does not usually result in clinical bleeding in the first six months of life. When hemophilia is severe and bleeding does occur, it is usually in the deep soft tissues or joints. Routine coagulation studies will be abnormal in the majority of cases. With some of the less common coagulopathies, either a bleeding time must be performed or specific factors assayed. Liver disease causes bleeding only in advanced stages. One would expect to see additional manifestations of hepatic failure, such as poor growth, jaundice, and/or hepatomegaly.

2. Since child abuse is the most likely diagnosis, you should file a report of suspected abuse with the child protective service. A skeletal survey may be ordered in an attempt to substantiate your impression, but the cutaneous findings are sufficient to initiate a report and normal X-rays would not invalidate your concerns about abuse. Skin biopsy is indicated in the evaluation for Ehlers Danlos syndrome, PT and PTT for hemophilia, and liver enzymes for hepatic disease.

Further Discussion

The manifestations of child abuse may be subtle, and the diagnosis, difficult to make. More than one million children are abused each year in the United States. Thus, the index of suspicion should remain high. The history of any injury, the physical findings, laboratory studies and X-rays, and observations of the parents must all be taken into consideration in reaching a conclusion about suspected abuse. A completely airtight case is not the standard for filing a report. Almost any bruising on a baby in the first 5-6 months of life is worthy of investigation.

Note that this infant has a Mongolian spot at the base of the spine; this is a normal variant that should not be confused with a bruise.

The parent of an 8-day-old calls the infant's pediatrician and describes a red, warm, swollen area over the baby's collarbone. Assuming a fractured clavicle, the nurse in the office recommends a visit the following morning. When the infant arrives, he is irritable with the following vital signs: P 140/min, R 38/min, BP 80/60 mm Hg, and T 37.9°C. The remainder of the examination is normal.

1. Based on the findings, you would
   A. Perform a complete sepsis evaluation
   B. Prescribe oral antibiotics
   C. Perform an aspiration and await cultures
   D. Apply a figure-of-eight dressing
   E. Draw HIV titers

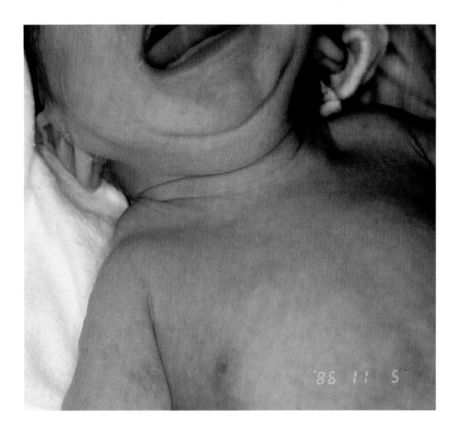

DISCUSSION

ANSWER:

1. **A. Perform a complete sepsis evaluation**

1. The swelling represents a supraclavicular adenitis. In any infant in the first month or two of life with a focal infection, even without a fever, a full evaluation for sepsis is necessary. In the absence of an inherited or acquired immunodeficiency, newborns are more susceptible to infection than older children and adults. Thus, HIV titers would not be indicated based on a single episode of adenitis and, furthermore, would not be a priority at this stage. Although aspiration of the node is important, it would not take priority over an evaluation for sepsis, including a lumbar puncture. Additionally, broad spectrum antibiotics are indicated prior to culture results. Oral antibiotic therapy is not sufficient for a focal infection at this age.

Further Discussion

An aspirate from the node, an aspirate from a swollen wrist not pictured here, and a culture of the blood grew Group B streptococci. Thus, this infant had Group B streptococcal sepsis, septic arthritis, and lymphadenitis. He recovered uneventfully, despite the delay in seeking care. This case makes three points. First, be wary of making diagnoses over the telephone. Second, with a few exceptions, never assume that an infection is focal in the first month of life. And third, the neonate does not always mount a febrile response to severe infection.

CASE 153

A 10-year-old male presents with joint pains for the last week. His parents recall removing a tick during a New England vacation 2 months ago.

1. If prompted, what type of rash might the parents recall their son having during the last 2 months?
   A. Ulcerations of the oral cavity
   B. A round lesion on the arm with central clearing
   C. A petechial rash on the wrist and ankles
   D. An evanescent salmon pink macular rash on the trunk
   E. A diffuse urticarial eruption

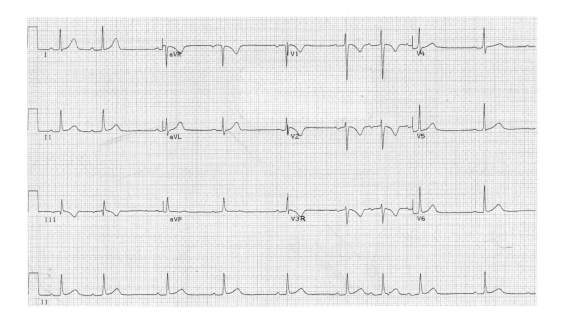

DISCUSSION

ANSWER:

1. **B. A round lesion on the arm with central clearing**

The EKG tracing shows sinus arrhythmia, sinus bradycardia, first degree heart block (a 10-year-old should have a PR interval of $< .17$) and type 1 second degree (Wenckebach) atrioventricular block. First degree heart block may be seen in healthy children or associated with myocarditis, some forms of congenital heart disease (atrial septal defects and Ebstein's anomaly), digitalis toxicity, acute rheumatic fever or with Lyme disease. The rash associated with Lyme disease, erythema chronicum migrans, is usually a red annular lesion expanding to greater than 5 cm. The center may clear. The annular lesion may began as a red papule at the site of the bite. This papule may blister or necrose. Between 70 and 80% of pediatric Lyme disease cases have erythema chronicum migrans.

Ulcerative lesions in the mouth occur with herpes simplex. Rocky Mountain spotted fever causes a petechial rash on the wrist and ankles; however, these patients also have fevers and headaches and deteriorate rapidly without therapy. An evanescent salmon pink macular rash might be seen on the trunk in systemic onset juvenile rheumatoid arthritis, often associated with fever, adenopathy and severe joint pain. Neither Rocky Mountain spotted fever nor juvenile rheumatoid arthritis is associated with first degree heart block.

Further Discussion

Lyme disease is quite common in certain areas of the country. Among the protean manifestations are fever, rash, Bell's palsy, aseptic meningitis, and myocarditis. Arising even more frequently than Lyme disease is the question of prophylaxis following tick bite. The only prospective study to date has not shown a statistically significant reduction in illness. On the other side of the equation, cases of Lyme disease occurred in the placebo but not the treatment group in the prospective study and a separate cost-benefit analysis favored prophylaxis in geographic regions where the prevalence of infected *Ixodes scapularis* was high. The final answer is not yet in.

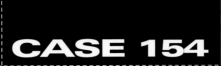

A 16-year-old previously healthy boy complains of scrotal pain. His general examination is normal.

1. After treating his acute problem, you order:
    A. A psychiatric consult
    B. A testicular scan
    C. A urologic consult
    D. A sperm count
    E. A urinalysis

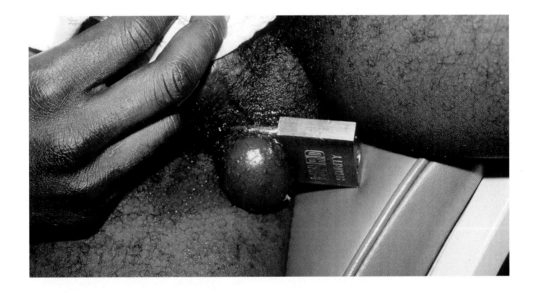

DISCUSSION

ANSWER:

1. **B. A testicular scan**

1. This young man stated he was "fooling around" with his girlfriend, when they realized that they did not have the key to this lock. Although some of you may consider this behavior quite atypical, it does not reach the level necessitating psychiatric consultation. Once you remove the lock, borrowing the proper tool from the maintenance department (see figure below), a urologist will not be of any assistance. Given that the impingement did not involve the penis or urethra, a urinalysis will be normal. A sperm count is unlikely to change with an acute insult and, even with complete failure of one testicle, may remain normal. Perhaps one could argue that no additional evaluation is needed, but vascular injury from compression may potentially lead to subsequent ischemic necrosis in the ensuing hours. Thus, a testicular scan was obtained, which proved to be normal.

Further Discussion

In the opinion of the editors, this case brings home the excitement experienced by those physicians in pediatrics, emergency medicine, and various other disciplines, who must be prepared to deal with the next child who walks through the door, no matter what the complaint. Additionally, it shows once again that a picture, without question (or in the case of this book, with questions) is worth a thousand words.

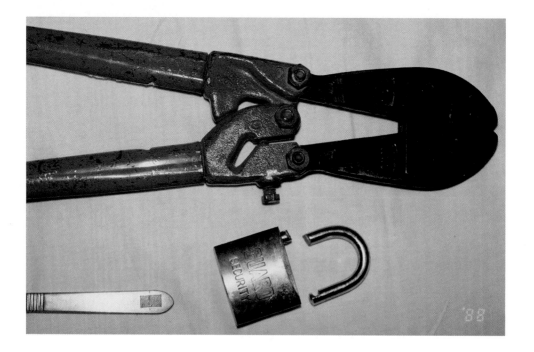

CASE LOCATOR

LIFE-THREATENING EMERGENCIES

Pediatric Resuscitation

Neonatal Resuscitation

Shock

Airway Management

SIGNS AND SYMPTOMS

Limp

Lymphadenopathy

Neck Mass

Neck Stiffness

Oligomenorrhea

Pain-Abdomen

Pain-Chest

Pain-Dysphagia

Pain-Dysuria

Pain-Headache

Pain Joints

Pain-Scrotal

Pallor

Rash-Eczematous

Rash-Papulosquamous

Rash-Purpura

MEDICAL EMERGENCIES

Cardiac Emergencies

Neurologic Emergencies

Infectious Disease Emergencies

Renal and Electrolyte Emergencies

Hematologic Emergencies

Toxicologic Emergencies

Environmental Emergencies

Bites and Stings

Allergic Emergencies

Pulmonary Emergencies

Gastrointestinal Emergencies

Pediatric and Adolescent Gynecology

Endocrine Emergencies

Metabolic Emergencies

Dermatology

Oncologic Emergencies

Rheumatologic Emergencies

TRAUMA

Approach to the Injured Child

Major Trauma

Head Trauma

Neck Trauma

Thoracic Trauma

Abdominal Trauma

Genitourinary Trauma

Thoracic Surgical Emergencies

Ophthalmologic Emergencies

Otolaryngology Emergencies

Urologic Emergencies

Orthopedic Emergencies

CASE LISTING

INDEX

Note: Page numbers in **boldface** indicate answers to questions.

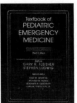
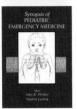
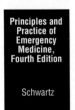
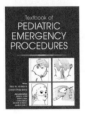
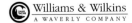